PSYCHIATRY AND THE MENTAL HEALTH PROFESSIONALS

New Roles for Changing Times

Report No. 122

PSYCHIATRY AND THE MENTAL HEALTH PROFESSIONALS

New Roles for Changing Times

Formulated by the
Committee on Governmental Agencies

Group for the Advancement of Psychiatry

BRUNNER/MAZEL *Publishers* • New York

Library of Congress Cataloging-in-Publication Data

Group for the Advancement of Psychiatry. Committee on
    Governmental Agencies.
    Psychiatry and the mental health professionals.

    (Report; no. 122)
    Includes bibliographies and index.
    1. Psychiatry.   2. Mental health.   I. Title.
II. Series: Report (Group for the Advancement of
Psychiatry); no. 122. [DNLM: 1. Mental Health Services
—manpower—United States.   2. Mental Health Services—
trends—United States.   3. Psychiatry—manpower—United
States.   4. Psychiatry—trends—United States.
W1 RE290BR no. 122 / WM 21 G882p]
RC321.G7 no. 122   [RC454]   616.89 s [362.2]   87-14588
ISBN 0-87630-474-9
ISBN 0-87630-473-0 (soft)

Copyright © 1987 by the Group for the Advancement of Psychiatry

Published by
BRUNNER/MAZEL, INC.
19 Union Square
New York, New York 10003

MANUFACTURED IN THE UNITED STATES OF AMERICA

10   9   8   7   6   5   4   3   2   1

STATEMENT OF PURPOSE

THE GROUP FOR THE ADVANCEMENT OF PSYCHIATRY has a membership of approximately 300 psychiatrists, most of whom are organized in the form of a number of working committees. These committees direct their efforts toward the study of various aspects of psychiatry and the application of this knowledge to the fields of mental health and human relations.

Collaboration with specialists in other disciplines has been and is one of GAP's working principles. Since the formation of GAP in 1946 its members have worked closely with such other specialists as anthropologists, biologists, economists, statisticians, educators, lawyers, nurses, psychologists, sociologists, social workers, and experts in mass communication, philosophy, and semantics. GAP envisages a continuing program of work according to the following aims:

1. To collect and appraise significant data in the fields of psychiatry, mental health, and human relations;
2. To reevaluate old concepts and to develop and test new ones;
3. To apply the knowledge thus obtained for the promotion of mental health and good human relations.

GAP is an independent group, and its reports represent the composite findings and opinions of its members only, guided by its many consultants.

PSYCHIATRY AND THE MENTAL HEALTH PROFESSIONALS: NEW ROLES FOR CHANGING TIMES was formulated by the Committee on Governmental Agencies. The members of this committee are listed on page vii. The members of the other GAP committees, as well as additional membership categories and current and past officers of GAP, are listed on pp. 191–197.

v

CONTENTS

INTRODUCTION

Core Psychiatric Identity

New scientific knowledge about mental illness has created enthusiasm within psychiatry for a diverse, but clearly medical identity for psychiatrists. The core professional identity of a contemporary psychiatrist is that of a physician who has acquired specialized knowledge regarding disorders affecting behavior and the mind. The psychiatric physician is capable of assuming a medical sense of responsibility for the treatment of his or her patients and is especially skillful in forming, analyzing, and maintaining the physician-patient relationship in a therapeutic alliance with the patient. In addition, the psychiatric physician must have comprehensive knowledge of diagnosis and treatment planning involving the use and *integration* of psychodynamic, pharmacological and social treatment modalities. Many psychiatrists may have additional special expertise in one area or another, whether it be in psychoanalysis or psychopharmacology, yet it is the advanced and sophisticated integrative competence described above that we believe patients must be able to assume is present when they consult a psychiatrist. A psychiatrist is a physician who is charged with seeing beyond mind/body dualism to a more fundamental living unity.

Comprehensive Diagnosis and Integrative Treatment Planning

The old medical adage that diagnosis is the crucial first step in the treatment of illness is increasingly true for mental illness as well.

Correct diagnosis, based on careful and comprehensive applications of differential diagnostic thinking, can be lifesaving.

As a result of their training, psychiatrists have diagnostic resources at their command by reason of medical training and clinical experience available to no other group, either medical or nonmedical. This diagnostic awareness can be crucial, for example, by preventing unnecessary surgery on a patient who experiences anxiety as abdominal pain, or by recognizing early signs of cardiac disease in a patient who might otherwise be thought to be only depressed. This is an area where we believe all psychiatrists bear a special obligation to remain current and comprehensive.

Treatment should follow from diagnostic and prognostic knowledge concerning the patient's illness, not from the fact that a given practitioner is only comfortable with a certain technique. A full survey of treatment options should be conducted and discussed with the patient. Of special importance is the capacity to use combined treatments together where this is indicated. For instance, in psychotherapy for depression, crucial benefits may accrue to the patient if antidepressant medication is added. Conversely, pharmacological treatment may not succeed for some patients without skilled and intensive psychotherapy. Attention to social supports may also be vital alongside psychotherapeutic and psychopharmacological intervention in treating other patients.

No Generic Mental Health Professional

Among the problems our patients face in seeking effective treatments are outdated roles for the care-giving professionals. The generic "mental health professional" is no longer a useful model. Psychiatrists are crucially distinct from general physicians, psychologists, social workers, and nurses by reason of length, depth, and breadth of clinical training in the care of the mentally ill. No other nonmedical group is equipped to accept the ultimate responsibility for the understanding and treatment of the mentally ill that psychiatrists have traditionally assumed. No other group is equipped to consider the diagnosis and treatment of mentally ill persons in such integrative depth. The mentally ill need nurses, psychologists, and social workers, as well as psychiatrists (and many other care givers), but they also need to understand the differences among the professionals to whom they turn for help.

New Knowledge

New knowledge that affects the treatment of the mentally ill is being generated at a great pace. Nosology has changed, although there is still significant debate in that area. There are new biological as well as psychodynamic dimensions of understanding of virtually all mental illnesses. Areas such as psychopharmacology, genetics, and neurophysiological investigation are in critical ferment. In addition, new social and psychodynamic understandings of developmental issues, of the impact of trauma on individuals and their families, and of relapse in the schizophrenias and affective disorders, all seem to have promise. The critical assimilation and thorough practical testing of new knowledge and hypotheses is a task that will require dedication and open-mindedness from all practitioners. Quality of care crucially depends on the ability to test new knowledge and to integrate its use in clinical treatment. Knowing the consequences to the profession and to our patients of excessive enthusiasm in the past decades, we must be cautioned to move with the data— not ahead of it.

About the Report

This Report by the Committee on Governmental Agencies of the Group for the Advancement of Psychiatry deals with some of the forces that will shape psychiatry's future, and with the impact of these forces on the relationships between psychiatrists and other professionals, both medical and nonmedical, who are involved with the care of people suffering from a mental illness. Our effort to peer into the future comes at a time of changing national priorities and new limitations on all health care funding. We hope that, by stating our views openly and assertively, we can generate active, informed discussion of the future treatment of the mentally ill and of the professional roles and relationships involved in such care, particularly as it relates to psychiatrists.

This Report is addressed to practitioners, mental health educators, legislators, and health care planners for industry and government in order to enhance their understanding of the needs of our patients. It points to changes that are necessary in the roles of psychiatrists and in relationships among all those who treat the mentally ill.

Our first chapter summarizes the development of psychiatry and the mental health movement, along with the growth of available manpower and its distribution and functions in various settings within the mental health arena. The second chapter introduces problems that have developed, due in part to an earlier excessive enthusiasm about our theories and capabilities, and in part to more recent economic pressures on the health care system as a whole.

The next chapters focus on those who provide treatment for the mentally ill, starting with a description of the profession of psychiatry— its basic tenets, the training required, unique characteristics, and relations with other disciplines. We include a chapter on the primary care system because of the sheer size of its contribution and conclude that a new, closer, and more helpful relationship with our medical colleagues is needed if we wish to address the needs of the mentally ill. Chapter 5 summarizes unresolved problems regarding our relations with other professionals and threats to our professional autonomy that come from the recent social and economic changes in our country that are revolutionizing all health care. We also discuss the precarious nature of third-party funding for psychotherapy.

Our final focus is on the explosion of new knowledge and perspectives that are affecting psychiatric theory and practice, and on implications for changes in the roles of psychiatrists that are suggested by the earlier chapters. In particular, we recommend development of "primary" and "subspecialized" roles for psychiatrists.

Since public opinion and public policy will be shaped by many forces with interests and perspectives other than our own, we invited representatives from clinical psychology, clinical social work, and psychiatric/mental health nursing to participate as independent consultants to our Committee. The resulting lively discussions modified our thinking in some areas to bring us into closer agreement and in other areas pointed up some sharp disagreements. A chapter from each consultant expressing that consultant's view of his or her own profession and positions disagreeing with the conclusion of our committee is appended to this *Report. While we emphasize that some of the opinions expressed in the Appendices are not endorsed by the Committee or by GAP,* we felt it important to include the views of spokesmen for other mental health disciplines, even if they differ from our own. Their inclusion should help the reader understand how psychiatry is different from other disciplines, how it is viewed by them, and how others see the development of their own disciplines.

PSYCHIATRY AND THE MENTAL HEALTH PROFESSIONALS

New Roles for Changing Times

Section 1

THE MENTAL HEALTH FIELD

1

AN OVERVIEW OF TODAY'S MENTAL HEALTH SERVICES

Origins and Growth of Today's Mental Health Professionals

Background

For centuries physicians have been called upon to treat persons who were thought to be mentally deranged depending to some extent on whether the culture of the times perceived these people as "sick," "wicked," or "possessed." In this country the first psychiatrists were general physicians like Benjamin Rush, a signer of the Declaration of Independence, who became interested in treating patients who suffered from mental illness. With a growing population and the creation of private and state mental hospitals in the nineteenth century, more physicians became involved with the mentally ill and, by 1844, developed psychiatry into a recognized specialty of medicine (Kolb & Brodie, 1982).

Clinical psychology developed gradually out of academic psychology in the late 1800s and became involved first in the mental health movement, and only later in the direct treatment of the mentally ill (Riesman, 1966).

Social work as an occupation in the United States began as early as the colonial days with the formalized establishment of public or private agencies to respond to community needs. Social work as a profession is largely a product of the mid-nineteenth and early twentieth centuries with the adoption of a body of knowledge, a technique (casework), and a professional association (The National Social Workers Exchange in 1917). Social workers did not begin to surface as specialists in mental health until early this century (Kohs, 1966).

Nursing, with its roots in the nineteenth century and even earlier (Appendix C), gradually became professionalized during the twentieth century and gained entrance into the mental health/illness field through public and private psychiatric hospitals. Only recently, as nurses raised their educational standards, did they become involved in mental health clinics and in private practice.

The mental health movement was founded in this country a year after the publication of Clifford Beers's *A Mind That Found Itself* in 1908 by the formation of the National Committee for Mental Hygiene (Beers, 1944). The early thrust of this movement was not directed toward the betterment of the mentally ill in our many large asylums, but toward creating a network of child guidance clinics aimed at preventing mental illness through parental education. This concept cited recognition of psychogenic determination in what had formerly been considered a medical or even spiritual problem.

Adolph Meyer, an outstanding leader in psychiatric education during the early part of this century, was to influence American psychiatry by emphasizing the effect of the social and interpersonal environment on each developing individual. He was a leader, along with Elmer Ernest Southard of the Boston Psychopathic Hospital, in encouraging social workers to play a major role in psychiatric treatment. Freud's psychoanalytic formulations were introduced from Europe early in this century, as well as those of Jung, Adler, Rank, and others. However, psychoanalysis did not become a major influence in clinics and in the private sector in this country until the late 1930s when many skilled psychiatrists, psychologists, and psychoanalysts escaped from Hitler's Europe to this country.

With a few notable exceptions, the mainstream of American psychiatry was primarily located in private and state psychiatric hospitals until after the end of World War II. Psychiatry was characterized by the limited, but sometimes successful use of sedative drugs and somatic treatments such as insulin or electroshock therapy, psychosurgery, and hydrotherapy. A merger of this mainstream of psychiatry, psychoanalysis, and the mental health movement took place in the late 1940s when the large number of psychiatric casualties associated with World War II became widely noted by the lay public. Leaders in psychiatry, especially psychoanalysts, gained congressional support to train thousands of psychiatrists in biologic, dynamic, and social theories during this period. In fact, the Group for the Advancement of Psychiatry was born in 1947 as an attempt to spread the new and exciting psychosocial and psychodynamic ideas to existing leaders of American psychiatry, as well as to interested people in other professions concerned with human affairs.

The potential for making effective changes appeared not only in the field of mental illness, but also in child rearing, education, criminology, national and international politics, and sociology. It appeared obvious that vast numbers of experts in mental health (not only mental illness) were needed in our growing, thriving, postwar society. In the late 1950s and early 1960s, our country's leaders perceived us as rich, expanding, powerful, and able to do anything we chose. It was in this context that psychiatric leaders, and eventually the U.S. Congress, embarked on a national program to provide mental health centers in each community. These were meant not only to treat the mentally ill, but also to try to prevent mental illness through community-oriented social and educational approaches (Caplan, 1964). Additional funds from the Congress were forthcoming to recruit and train an expanded work force of mental health professionals. Both the organized mental health systems and, with the growing availability of third-party medical insurance, the private practice sector grew to meet the available funding and the increased expectations of the public.

Psychiatrists, along with other mental health professionals, began to identify themselves as generic "mental health professionals," rather than as members of distinct disciplines with unique skills. New medications enabled the long-term mentally ill to benefit from social and psychological services and many became well enough to go home. State hospitals were emptied across the nation by moving their better patients back to hometown communities, with the expectation that the newly promised community mental health centers (CMHCs) would provide follow-up treatment. The acceptance of the concept of "entitlement" to mental and other health care paralleled this movement. Although there were still problems to be worked out, there seemed to be enough ideas and money and mental health professionals to provide mental health for all. It looked as if, finally, hopes for spreading the benefits of mental health knowledge throughout our society could be achieved.

In the next chapter we will address a variety of realities that blunted this dream. It is important to note the stark contrast between the political climate in the 1960s and early 1970s and that of today, where there is a national mandate to cut governmental spending, particularly in the health and welfare sector. Today, also, community mental health programs and psychiatric treatment in general tend to be considered by the government, insurance carriers, unions, much of the public, and even by many professionals as a low-yield, low-priority, high-cost luxury (Group for the Advancement of Psychiatry, 1983).

Numbers and Distribution of Mental Health Professionals

In 1950 there were only 7,100 psychiatrists and child psychiatrists, 7,300 psychologists belonging to the American Psychological Association (few of them clinicians), approximately 9,500 clinical social workers, and virtually no psychiatric nurses (Arnhoff, Rubinstein, Shriver, & Jones, 1969). The interest in mental health that followed the Second World War has led to a far different picture today.

Psychiatry. In 1981 the American Medical Association (Eiler, 1983) reported that there were 28,524 psychiatrists and 3,295 child psychiatrists, for a total of 31,819, or a rate of 14.0 per 100,000 population. That year 89% (28,250) of all psychiatrists cited patient care as their major professional activity, and 59% (18,913) were primarily in office-based practice. Far more than is the case with nonpsychiatric physicians, psychiatrists are members of the full-time physician staff of facilities (5,677 or 18%) or list administration as their primary activity (1,966 or 6%). This difference is undoubtedly a reflection of the large public mental health system. Note that there were 22,565 filled psychiatric positions in public and private mental health facilities in the United States in 1978 to make up 14,492 full-time equivalent positions (NIMH, unpublished data, 1978). Psychiatrists are very likely to have more than one work setting and to do some private practice.

Like most specialists, psychiatrists are unevenly distributed geographically across the country and are located predominantly in urbanized areas and states (Eiler, 1983). Four states (Massachusetts, New York, Connecticut, and Maryland) have a rate of over 20 nonfederal psychiatrists per 100,000 civilian population, compared to a national average of 13.2. The District of Columbia, which should properly be compared to cities not states, has a ratio of 64.8. At the other extreme, six states (Wyoming, Idaho, South Dakota, Montana, Alaska, and Mississippi) have less than five psychiatrists per 100,000 civilian population.

Psychology. The exact number of clinical psychologists is unknown. In 1980 there were 49,085 members of the American Psychological Association, which estimates that 90% of doctoral psychologists belong to this organization. Only a fraction of those trained at the master's level are members.

In 1980 there were 21.7 American Psychological Association member psychologists per 100,000 population (VandenBos, Stapp, & Kilbury, 1981). Four states and the District of Columbia have a rate of more than 30 American Psychological Association members per 100,000 population. These are the same states that have an abundant supply of psychiatrists. Arkansas, Kentucky, Louisiana, and Mississippi have less than 10 American Psychological Association members per 100,000 population.

Not all psychologists are trained to provide health or mental health services, although 60% of respondents to a 1978 American Psychological Association survey indicated that they were engaged in this activity to some extent. Counting members as well as nonmembers, there may be as many as 35,000 service-provider psychologists, approximately half of them spending 20 hours a week or less in clinical work. The doctoral degree is widely recognized as necessary for independent practice, and the great majority of master's level psychologists work in organized care settings or in schools. About 45% of the doctoral health-service-provider psychologists list private practice as their primary service delivery setting, but, because this is a part-time activity for many, only 25% have private practice as their primary employment setting.

Social work. In 1981 there were 86,757 members of the National Association of Social Workers (NASW) residing in the United States, or a rate of 37.7 per 100,000 population. This reflects a growth of 231% since 1960 (NASW, 1960–1981). The Association estimates that 70%–80% of all active social workers trained at the master's level are members, but many individuals who are educated at the bachelor's level or who occupy social work positions do not belong to the Association.

Social workers are trained generically, so it is difficult to state exactly how many can be defined as psychiatric specialists. A common estimate is that 25% of all social workers are primarily involved in mental health, but movement into and out of the field is common. Using this figure, there would be approximately 21,700 NASW member and 7,300 nonmember social workers in the mental health field. Since almost 10,000 individuals receive a master's degree in social work each year (Rubin, 1982), there is ample replenishment of the supply, and in fact there is some indication of an oversupply.

Social workers traditionally have worked in organized care settings for health, mental health, and social services, but in recent years greater numbers have engaged in private practice. The NASW Register of Clinical Social Workers (1982) can be used as an index of participation in this activity. In 1982, 8,733 social workers were listed on the Register, yielding a ratio of 3.8 per 100,000 population. As with psychologists and psychiatrists, the District of Columbia and the four states of New York, Massachusetts, Connecticut, and Maryland had proportionately the greatest concentration, with ratios of over twice the national average. Seventeen states, in the south, west-central, and Appalachian areas, had less than two registered clinical social workers per 100,000 population.

Psychiatric nursing. There were an estimated 1,119,100 registered nurses in the United States in 1980 (U.S. Department of Health and Human Services, 1981). Usually, about 5% identify psychiatric/mental health nursing as their area of clinical practice. Of the 51,564 who did so in the most recent (1977–78) *Inventory* (American Nurses' Association, 1981), almost two-thirds were trained at less than the baccalaureate level. Another 6,579, or 12.8%, had a master's or higher degree, although many of these degrees were in fields other than nursing.

Approximately 70% of all mental health nurses work in hospitals, and an additional 10.6% in community health, including mental health. Over 6% are employed in schools of nursing. Only 395, or less than 1%, state that they are "self-employed, other than private duty."

The distribution of employment is somewhat different for those psychiatric/mental health nurses with master's or higher degrees. Only 38% work in hospitals, while 36% are employed in schools of nursing and 12% in community health settings. Three percent are self-employed other than in private-duty nursing.

Psychiatric nursing has the highest proportion of nurses educated at the graduate level of any field in nursing (National League for Nursing, 1977). From 1965 through 1975 20%–25% of all master's degrees in nursing were in the psychiatric/mental health area. This percentage has since dropped, although the absolute number of degrees awarded in this field has continued to rise slowly. Nursing educators fear a drop in production and a future shortage of psychiatric nurses.

Scope of Organized Mental Health Settings

Mental health care is delivered in a wide variety of settings. The organized mental health care sector included 3,727 facilities in 1980, ranging from large state mental hospitals to small outpatient clinics. Their distribution and the type of services offered are shown in Table 1.1.

The number of state and county mental hospitals has decreased from 310 in 1970 to 280 in 1980 (Taube & Barrett, 1983), but the number of all other types of facilities has increased, with the exception of freestanding outpatient clinics. Most of the increase has been due to the growth of CMHCs.

State and county mental hospitals accounted for 57% of the 274,713 inpatient beds, 25% of the 1,541,659 inpatient admissions, and 30% of the 1,779,587 inpatient episodes in 1979–1980 (Taube & Barrett, 1983). In all categories this percentage has fallen since 1970, when 79% of the inpatient beds were in these facilities. In 1979, 32% of the inpatient episodes were in nonfederal general hospital psychiatric units, 14% were in CMHCs, 12% in Veterans Administration facilities, 9% in private psychiatric hospitals, and 3% in other facilities. The number of inpatient additions and episodes and the rate per 100,000 population decreased in 1979, probably reflecting a national effort to avoid hospitalization whenever possible. The average daily census and the number of inpatients at the end of the year have been declining steadily for a decade.

In contrast, the number of outpatient visits to all facilities (Taube & Barrett, 1983) has been growing rapidly, from 1,146,612 in 1969 to 2,634,727 in 1979. This latter figure reflects a rate of 1,188 per 100,000 civilian population. The great majority of these patients were seen in CMHCs (47%) or freestanding psychiatric outpatient clinics (31%). For all outpatient admissions the median number of visits for all diagnoses was 3.7, and in no category did the number of visits exceed 4.5 (NIMH, unpublished data, 1975). Only 14% of admissions were seen for more than 10 visits, and only in the category of schizophrenia were more than 5% of the patients seen for more than 20 visits.

As might be expected, state and county mental hospitals have a resident population composed largely of patients with the chronic disabilities of schizophrenia, organic brain syndrome, and mental retardation (Taube & Barrett, 1983; NIMH, unpublished data,

Table 1.1*

Number of Mental Health Facilities in the U.S. in 1980
by Type of Facility and Type of Service

All Facilities	Total	Number of Mental Health Facilities		
		With Inpatient Services	With Outpatient Services	With Day Treatment Services
State and county mental hospitals	280	280	100	83
Private psychiatric hospitals	184	184	54	68
Nonfederal general hospitals with separate psychiatric services	923	843	299	165
Veterans Administration psychiatric services	136	121	127	67
Federally funded community mental health centers	691	691[a]	691	691
Residential treatment centers for emotionally disturbed children	368	368	68	104
Freestanding psychiatric outpatient clinics	1,053	—	1,053	381
All other facilities	92	39	39	89
Total, all facilities	3,727	2,526	2,431	1,648

*Adapted from Taube and Barrett, 1983, pp. 10–14, Tables 2.1a–2.1d.

[a]Many of the inpatient CMHC services are contracted with other facilities already on this table, thus there is some duplication.

1975). New patients tend to be suffering from schizophrenia, alcohol or drug disorders, or depression. Short-stay nonfederal hospitals, in contrast, see proportionally more patients with alcohol or drug disorders, depression and affective disorders, and neuroses. Outpatient facilities see proportionally fewer patients with psychoses or substance abuse problems and more with neuroses, personality disorders, transient situational disorders, and social maladjustment problems. CMHCs, which contain both inpatient and outpatient units, tend to fall between these extremes.

Other specialized mental health settings include college campus mental health clinics and the offices of mental health private practitioners, which combined probably treat almost 1.5 million persons.

Regier, Goldberg, and Taube (1978) have estimated that only 21% of all persons with mental disorders are seen in the specialized mental health sector. They hypothesize that an additional 3.4% are seen in hospitals and nursing homes and 60% in the outpatient primary medical care sector. The remaining 21.5% are supposedly seen in the social services sector, the criminal justice system, or not seen at all. No data are available on the mental health care provided in social service agencies or on the number of people with mental disorders who seek support from self-help groups or voluntary agencies serving the poor, including the mentally ill.

Practice in Organized Mental Health Systems

Staff in organized systems are generally salaried, rather than paid on a fee-for-service basis, and are selected and supervised by a hierarchical administration that often imposes its own set of priorities. Characteristically, assignment of patients to staff tends to be done through an organized intake process, and service delivery tends to involve multidisciplinary teams.

Numbers and Distribution of the Providers

There were 430,051 full-time equivalent (FTE) staff in mental health facilities in the United States in 1978, with 292,699 categorized as performing patient care (Taube & Barrett, 1983). Of these, 101,517, or 35%, were members of one of the four core mental health disciplines of psychiatry, psychology, social work, and nursing (registered nurses only). Full-time equivalent staff working in these facilities accounted for approximately half of all psychiatrists and health-services-provider psychologists in the country at that time and 82% of the nurses who reported a clinical specialty of psychiatric/mental health nursing.

Not all of these professionals were fully trained. Approximately 25% of the psychiatrists were residents, and 52% of the psychologists did not have doctoral degrees. Twenty-four percent of the social workers had less than a master's degree. It can be estimated that over two-thirds of the nurses had less than a bachelor's degree and more than 90% had less than a master's degree.

The distribution of full-time equivalent professional staff in these disciplines among the types of mental health facilities is shown in Table 1.2.

It can be seen that psychiatrists and nurses are most often on the staff of inpatient facilities, especially state and county mental hospitals and the psychiatric units of nonfederal general hospitals. In contrast, social workers and psychologists are most heavily concentrated in freestanding outpatient clinics and community mental health centers. Many are also found in state and county mental hospitals, as these institutions overall employ 31% of the FTE professional patient-care staff in all facilities.

The composition of patient-care staff in mental health facilities has been changing over the years. On the one hand it has become more professional, with the proportion of FTE staff who are licensed practical or vocational nurses, or mental health workers with less than a baccalaureate degree, declining from 50% to 42% between 1972 and 1978. On the other hand, the growth has been for the most part in the category of "other mental health professional, BA and above," where the number of FTE staff has risen by 125% in the six-year period. Comparable growth figures for the professions are psychiatry, 12%; psychology, 75%; social work, 59%; and registered nurses, 36% (Taube & Barrett, 1983).

Table 1.2*

Distribution of Full-Time Equivalent Professional Staff Positions in Mental Health
Facilities in the United States, by Discipline and Type of Facility, 1978

Type of Facility	Discipline								Total
	Psychiatrists		Psychologists		Social Workers		Registered Nurses		
	N	%	N	%	N	%	N	%	N
State and county mental hospitals	3,712	26	3,149	19	5,924	21	14,859	35	27,644
Private mental hospitals	1,285	9	590	4	920	3	3,967	9	9,762
Veterans Administration psychiatric services	1,745	12	1,392	8	1,611	6	5,814	14	10,562
Nonfederal general hospital psychiatric services	3,583	25	1,512	9	2,552	9	10,611	25	18,258
Residential treatment centers	140	1	497	3	2,196	8	324	1	3,157
Freestanding outpatient clinics	1,413	10	4,115	25	6,513	23	882	2	12,923
Federally funded community mental health centers	2,246	15	4,796	29	7,329	26	5,469	13	19,840
Others	368	2	450	3	1,080	4	473	1	2,371
Total	14,492	100	16.501	100	28,125	100	42,399	100	101,517

*Adapted from Taube and Barrett, 1983, pp. 132–134, Table 5.24.

During the 1970s, while the actual number of psychiatrists and other physicians on the staff of mental health facilities increased in all settings except for state and county mental hospitals, the proportion of patient-care staff who were psychiatrists decreased during that period except in VA psychiatric settings. This decrease is most noticeable in freestanding outpatient clinics (50%), private psychiatric hospitals (33%), CMHCs (31%), and nonfederal general hospitals (22%). The number of FTE psychiatrists working in mental health facilities actually declined 5.5% between 1976 and 1978 (Taube & Barrett, 1983).

In part the new staff are well-qualified psychologists, social workers, and nurses, but all too often budget considerations lead facilities to hire staff that have not been fully trained in any discipline. The effect that this is having on patient care has not been adequately studied.

Staffing Patterns Within Settings

The GAP Committee on Governmental Agencies studied manpower utilization in samples of four organized mental health settings (see Table 1.3). Distinct staffing patterns emerged from the Committee's study of the literature describing CMHCs (Task Panel

Table 1.3
Staff Distribution Within Sample
Organized Mental Health Settings

	CMHCs	HMOs	VAPCs	GEN HOSPs
Psychiatrists	6.4	26.0	15.0	10.2
Psychologists	12.7	22.0	8.0	8.1
Social workers	18.9	47.0	7.0	7.0
Registered nurses	12.9	4.0	26.0	36.0
Others, B.A. level	17.8	—	—	5.6
Paraprofessionals	26.0	1.0	34.0	33.1
Others	5.3	—	10.0	—
Total	100.0%	100.0%	100.0%	100.0%

on Mental Health Personnel, 1978), an informal survey of five closed-staff health maintenance organization (HMO) (Sidney Goldensohn, personal communication, February 1980)* reports regarding Veterans Administration psychiatric centers (VAPCs) (Administrator of Veterans Affairs, 1978), and a survey of psychiatric directors of six general medical hospitals in New England (James P. Cattell, personal communication, November 8, 1979).†

Both CMHCs and HMOs are primarily outpatient oriented, yet the CMHC data are striking in that the four core disciplines represent only a bare majority (50.9%) of the staff involved in direct patient care. Furthermore, a study by the National Council of Community Mental Health Centers, Inc. (1979), reveals that this core group provided only 37.5% of total hours of patient care, leaving one to speculate that a large percentage of direct patient care in this system is handled by staff whose qualifications would be considered marginal.

A survey of staff utilization in eight CMHCs in 1968 (Glasscote & Gudeman, 1969) revealed the enormous differences between centers that are obscured in pooled statistical data. Psychiatrists ranged from 5%-29% of all staff, psychologists from 5%-15%, social workers from 11%-47%, nurses from 4%-24% and mental health aides from 7%-42%.

Functions of the Providers

Our survey of general hospital psychiatric inpatient services was limited to inquiry about the various disciplines' participation in either individual, group, or family psychotherapies, in evaluation of the effects of medication, in emergency room screenings, in liaison and consultation, or in supervision by or of other disci-

---

*Survey included Kaiser Plan of Los Angeles, Kaiser Plan of San Francisco, Harvard Community Health Plan of Cambridge and Boston, Massachusetts, Marshfield Clinic of Marshfield, Wisconsin, and Health Insurance Plan of New York, 1980.

†Survey included Framingham Union Hospital, Framingham, MA; University of Massachusetts Medical Center, Worchester, MA; Eastspoke, Franklin County Public Hospital, Greenfield, MA; Berkshire Medical Center, Pittsfield, MA; Baystate Medical Center, Springfield, MA; State University Hospital, Downstate Medical Center, Brooklyn, N.Y.

plines. The functions of our sample of core mental health professionals vary widely, from each discipline participating in all functions surveyed to being active in none.

The psychiatrist has the ultimate professional and legal responsibility for the care of psychiatric patients in the general hospital. This responsibility includes an initial evaluation and official diagnosis, although members of other disciplines often provide significant input of clinical data.

The psychologists with doctorate degrees are next in line with regard to authority and influence. They are involved in all of the psychotherapies and many are involved in providing supervision. They consult on patients in the emergency room in all hospitals except one, where this responsibility is restricted to the psychiatrists. They provide consultation services to medical/surgical areas in only three of the hospitals.

In addition to more traditional duties, social workers provide all psychotherapies in two general hospital settings, family therapy and emergency room consultation in one, and consultation to medical/surgical staff in two.

Nurses perform in all psychotherapies in four facilities, but are restricted to group therapy in one, and are not used in another. Paraprofessionals, all of whom have baccalaureate degrees or better in five of the six hospitals, are involved in all psychotherapies in those hospitals. The crucial job of monitoring both therapeutic and side effects of potent psychotropic medications is delegated essentially to all disciplines, but particularly to nurses and paraprofessionals, who spend most of their time with patients and are in a position to perceive subtle nuances and symptoms before they become dramatic. A similar wide variation in distribution of numbers and roles of mental health disciplines occurs in VA psychiatric settings (National Academy of Sciences National Research Council, 1977; Van Stone, 1978).

Our inquiry of five HMO clinics revealed that, in general, each staff member is expected to assume responsibility for the overall treatment of his patient regardless of his particular professional discipline, although medication is supervised by a psychiatrist.

Treatment is most likely carried out by a medical doctor when a patient has a complex medical problem or needs careful drug titration. Only the psychologist conducts testing evaluations (projective, intellectual, and educational). The psychiatric nurse/clinician is used more heavily for hospital liaison and emergency psychiatry, and the psychiatric social worker is additionally called on as a source of information about available community resources.

In a 1976 survey of training programs in 55 CMHCs in 13 western states (Bloom & Parad), 66% of respondents stated that "task responsibilities on teams were assigned on the basis of competence without regard to discipline" (p. 672), 85% noted shared responsibility for patients, 86% said the same for diagnosis of patients, 78% said that most decisions were made by team consensus, and 85% indicated that "contributions to team discussions were judged by merit rather than by disciplinary status" (p. 672). If truly representative, these findings suggest a low degree of functional differentiation in CHMCs.

In summary, the core mental health professionals have performed a wide range of mental health tasks, somewhat independent of professional background. A surprising finding is that the patterns of utilization vary widely from setting to setting, even within the same system.

Private Practice

Mental Health Professionals in Private Practice

Until recent years, psychiatrists were by far the predominant group in private practice. With changes in access to insurance reimbursement, stimulated primarily by clinical psychologists, the other groups have begun to enter private practice in increasing numbers. There are, for example, now approximately 19,000 psychiatrists, 10,000 psychologists, 3,000 licensed clinical social workers, and 300 master's-level psychiatric/mental health nurses in private practice.

The distribution of these practitioners tends to parallel the distribution of other elements in health care, with clustering in major urban areas. Many groups are underrepresented in the patient population of private practitioners, including the poor, the elderly, inner-city and rural residents, chronic schizophrenic patients, and substance abusers.

Psychiatrists tend to see the broadest range of patients, from the sickest to the healthiest, from all diagnostic categories, all ages, and all segments of society. They are involved in the full range of modalities including diagnosis, evaluation of medical/psychological interactions, a range of psychotherapies, prescription and monitoring of medications, crisis intervention, and consultation. They will usually treat patients in both outpatient and hospital settings, and assume responsibility for continuity of treatment through all phases of a patient's illness.

The private practice of psychologists tends to parallel that of psychiatrists in some but not all areas. They probably see few patients with major psychotic illness, fewer elderly patients, and fewer patients with mixed organic and psychological problems. They tend to use behavior therapies more often than psychiatrists and are trained to perform psychological testing. They do not prescribe medications nor, with recent exceptions, admit patients to hospitals, although they are presently gaining access to some hospital staffs. Psychologists are no longer required to maintain a routine relationship with a psychiatrist for evaluation of patients and treatment planning or supervision.

Social workers see many patients and use many forms of psychotherapy that overlap with the two groups already discussed. They see more people who present with family problems, and fewer with diagnostic problems or major illnesses. They use a broad range of psychotherapies, especially supportive therapy, couple and family therapy, and crisis intervention. Many social workers maintain an ongoing relationship with a psychiatrist, whom they consult for diagnostic and treatment supervision. The trend for social workers, however, like psychologists, is toward greater autonomy of practice.

Nurses in private practice are too few in number for assessment of trends. While it is possible that nurses in private practice may continue to see the population they have traditionally seen in hospitals and clinics—severely ill patients who need supportive psychotherapy and monitoring of medications under psychiatric supervision—it seems more likely that they will see private practices that parallel more closely those of social workers.

Advantages of Private Practice

The advantages of private practice, common to all the professional groups involved, include maximal autonomy for patients and for professionals and a minimum of bureaucratic interference with professional judgment and decision making.

The patient has the choice, when he enters the private practice system, of selecting the type of professional he wants to consult. He can use criteria of therapist age, sex, race, professional orientation, credentials, location, or personal recommendation from others. Assuming that the patient's initial level of confidence in the therapist may affect treatment outcome, this freedom to select the therapist may increase the probability that the treatment will be helpful. Similarly, the therapist's freedom to concentrate on certain types of treatment, patients, or problems may enable him to capitalize on his personal strengths.

A fee-for-service system, with the practitioners earning their income through hours spent in treating patients, tends to maximize productivity and minimize time spent on paperwork, meetings, and other nonearning functions. The demands of government for reporting, form-filling, etc., have entered the private practice system so far through private insurance, Medicaid, Medicare, and Champus. While this burden is growing rapidly, it is still smaller than the demands placed on institutions. Some feel that the minimization of record-keeping, statistical-reporting, and meetings may in fact be a drawback in private practice. Many practitioners, in fact, seek out part-time teaching or other affiliation with colleagues in order to discuss cases, to keep up with new thinking in their fields, and to combat the loneliness that is frequently mentioned as a drawback to private practice. On the whole, however, the freedom from institutional rules, the ability to answer only to the patient and to act in his interests, and the ability to assure confidentiality to the patient are generally seen as advantages.

Disadvantages of Private Practice

In general, it is the tendency of a private practitioner to treat any patient who seeks his or her help with the methods that he knows how to use, unless there is a glaring lack of fit between the patient's needs and the therapist's skills. Any single practitioner is usually more limited in his potential treatment methods than the full array of possible therapists may be able to provide. Pride, an unwillingness to be seen as admitting limitations on his skills, fear of "losing" the patient, economic motives, and interprofessional rivalries may all be factors in the relative unwillingness of the therapist in private practice to use the additional skills of others as readily as might happen in a clinic or other organized setting.

The most serious problems of private practice lie in the diagnosis and treatment-planning areas. Many psychiatrists believe that evaluation of a patient's problem requires the involvement of a psychiatrist in order to determine if the problem is a mental disorder and if it is best treated by psychotherapy, by medication, or by a combination of the two. The inappropriate prescription of psychotherapy by nonpsychiatrists when the problem is primarily caused by an endocrine or neurological illness, or the failure to use psychotropic medications for conditions where they have been shown to alter the course of psychiatric illness, can have serious negative consequences for the patient.

At present, while many social workers and nurses do maintain a relationship with a psychiatrist for diagnostic and consultation purposes, there is no requirement that they do so; indeed, many do not. Psychologists rarely maintain such a relationship with a psychiatrist, and generally disagree with the need for psychiatric involvement in the diagnostic process, especially with referrals from primary care physicians.

A related problem is the frequent lack in private practice of easy referral of patients to other practitioners for additional help. For example, a patient in psychotherapy with a social worker may not be referred to a psychologist for a brief course of behavior therapy, or a psychiatrist's patient may not be referred to a social worker for a course of conjoint therapy, when these additional treatments may be appropriate.

These drawbacks are all part of the larger problem of a lack, in private practice, of any system of triage. No one considers the relative severity of problems and allocates resources accordingly. The patient who arrives at each practitioner's door is treated as well as that professional can manage, with little real consideration of the marginal advantage to the patient of referral to another practitioner, and no consideration of the needs of the patients who did not arrive.

Governmental Influences on Mental Health Roles

Both federal and state governments have supported programs and developed regulations that have had a great influence on the roles, development, activities, and reimbursement of mental health professionals.

Federal Government

Training. Since the passage of the Mental Health Act in 1946, the Federal Government has been actively involved in the training and education of psychiatrists and other mental health professionals. Initially, support was given to improve the quality of training and increase the numbers of well-qualified practitioners in the four core disciplines. Training grants, along with programs administered by the Veterans Administration, were crucial in the establishment and improvement of academic departments and in providing the financial support that enabled students to complete their education. More recently, the National Institute of Mental Health (NIMH) has redirected its program to focus more on training practitioners to work with underserved population groups such

FOR REVIEW

PSYCHIATRY AND THE MENTAL
HEALTH PROFESSIONALS:
New Roles for Changing Times
(GAP Report No. 122)

Committee on
Governmental Agencies

PRICE: $13.95 (paper)
           $19.50 (cloth)

PAGES: 216

SIZE: 6 x 9

LCN#:   87-14588

ISBN#:   0-87630-473-0 (paper)
           0-87630-474-9 (cloth)

Publication Date: October 18, 1987

Please send two copies of your review to:
BRUNNER/MAZEL Publishers
19 Union Square, New York, N.Y. 10003
Tel.: (212) 924-3344

BOOKS IN PSYCHOANALYSIS / PSYCHIATRY / PSYCHOLOGY / CHILD DEVELOPMENT

as children, the elderly, and minorities and to accept employment in public facilities as well as rural or inner-city geographic areas. Federal programs have been effective in increasing the number of minority practitioners and in promoting innovations in education, such as consultation/liaison psychiatry, and community psychiatry and psychology.

Services. The massive federal investment in the establishment of CMHCs throughout the nation has made mental health services available to many who, before this development, could not afford them or would have been reluctant to seek professional help with their problems. At the same time, the emphasis on community involvement, case finding, and the social and psychosocial causes of many mental health problems led to a broadening of the definition of mental illness and brought large numbers of nonmedical practitioners and paraprofessional personnel onto the staff of CMHCs. This, in turn, fostered the growth of these disciplines and strengthened their role in the mental health service delivery system.

State Government

Licensure. The major function of individual states in regard to the mental health professions is that the states have the authority to license practitioners. Licensure may define and restrict the scope of practice of a profession or it may merely restrict the use of a title, so that untrained and unlicensed personnel may not call themselves psychologists or social workers when offering services to the public. In either case, licensure defines the members of a profession, theoretically assures a given quality or at least amount of education, and may help to raise the likelihood of competent services. Possession of a professional license also makes it easier to obtain third-party reimbursement, since the insurer knows that the number of eligible providers will be limited and that there is the presumption of quality. For this reason, psychologists and social workers sought to pass licensing laws in the states. Psychologists have been successfull in all 50 states and the District of Columbia, and social workers are licensed in 23 states. Many states, however, have begun to pass "sunset laws" under which these actions are periodically reexamined and sometimes allowed to lapse. Psychiatrists and psychiatric nurses are licensed generically as physician and nurses, respectively.

Other regulations. States may also pass laws that directly affect professional practice. Many states have "freedom-of-choice" laws that recognize psychologists or social workers as independent practitioners and mandate coverage for their services if similar services are covered when provided by other practitioners. The Supreme Court has ruled that insurance companies violate antitrust laws if they do not provide for direct reimbursement and instead attempt to require billing through a physician. There is considerable controversy among the mental health professionals over freedom of choice laws, with psychiatrists opposing them and the nonmedical disciplines favoring them.

Staffing of state-funded facilities. States hire staff and establish salary scales for many of the mental health facilities within their boundaries. Although few have developed any formal staffing standards as such, both the need for accreditation of facilities and the desire to provide care of a reasonable quality have meant that states have tried to maintain a certain level of qualified professional staff in the facilities over which they have control. As financial problems mount, however, staff may be laid off and there is an incentive to hire and retain lower level, less highly trained staff. Master's-level psychologists, bachelor's-level social workers, and nurses without a graduate degree may be preferred to their better qualified counterparts. This may impair not only the quality of service in the facility, but also inflict wider damage on the image and job opportunities of the profession as a whole.

In spite of recent rhetoric about deregulation, the activities of federal and state governments have a profound impact on the range of activities, employment opportunities, and income of all mental health professionals. In many cases their interests differ, and each profession seeks legislation to further its own interests. If too much acrimony is perceived by legislators and the public, it may in the end be the patient who suffers most when laws promoting access to mental health care of high quality are not enacted.

References

Administrator of Veterans Affairs. *Annual Report 1978* (p. 9). Washington, DC: U.S. Government Printing Office, 1978.

American Nurses' Association. *Inventory of Registered Nurses, 1977-78.* Kansas City, MO. Author, 1981.

Arnhoff, F.N., Rubinstein, E.A., Shriver, B.M., & Jones, D.R. The mental health fields: An overview of manpower growth and development (Chapter 1). In F.N. Arnhoff, E.A. Rubinstein, & J.C. Speisman (Eds.), *Manpower for Mental Health.* Chicago, Aldine: 1969.

Beers, C.W., *A Mind That Found Itself: An Autobiography* (6th ed.). New York: Doubleday, Doran, 1944. (Original work published 1908)

Bloom, B.L. & Parad H.J. Interdisciplinary training and interdisciplinary functioning: A survey of attitudes and practices in community mental health. *American Journal of Orthopsychiatry,* 46:669-676, 1976.

Caplan, G., *Principles of Preventive Psychiatry.* New York: Basic Books, 1964.

Eiler, M.A. *Physician Characteristics and Distribution in the U.S. (1982 ed.).* Chicago, IL: Division of Survey and Data Resources, American Medical Association, 1983.

Glasscote, R.M., & Gudeman, J.E. *The Staff of the Mental Health Center: A Field Study.* Washington, DC: Joint Information Service of the American Psychiatric Association and the National Association for Mental Health, 1969.

Group for the Advancement of Psychiatry. Committee on Psychiatry and the Community. *Community Psychiatry: A Reappraisal. Report No. 113* (Chapter 1). New York: Mental Health Materials Center, Inc., 1983.

Kohs, S.C. *The Roots of Social Work* (pp. 142, 148, 153). NY Association Press, 1966.

Kolb, L.C. & Brodie, K.H. *Modern Clinical Psychiatry* (Chapter 1) (10th ed.). W.B. Saunders 1982.

National Academy of Sciences National Research Council, *Study of Health Care for American Veterans* (pp. 89, 170, 181, 186). Washington, DC: U.S. Government Printing Office, June 7, 1977.

National Association of Social Workers. *Annual Report of Membership Statistics.* Silver Spring, MD: Author, 1960-1981.

National Association of Social Workers. *Register of Clinical Social Workers. 1982* (3rd ed.). Silver Spring, MD: Author, 1982.

National Council of Community Mental Health Centers, Inc. *Salary Survey.* Mimeo, March, 1979.

National Institute of Mental Health, Division of Biometry and Applied Sciences. Unpublished data, 1975.

National Institute of Mental Health. [Inventory of mental health facilities]. Unpublished data, 1978.

National League for Nursing. *Some Statistics on Baccalaureate and Higher Degree Education in Nursing, 1977.* New York, NY: Author, 1977.

Regier, D.A., Goldberg, I.D., & Taube, C.A. The de facto U.S. mental health services system. *Archives of General Psychiatry,* 35:685–693, 1978.

Riesman, J.M. *The Development of Clinical Psychology,* East Norwalk, CT: Appleton-Century-Crofts, 1966.

Rubin, A. (Ed.). *Statistics on Social Work Education in the United States: 1981.* New York, NY: Council on Social Work Education, 1982.

Task Panel on Mental Health Personnel. *Task Panel Reports, Vol. II* (appendix; p. 485). Submitted to the President's Commission on Mental Health, Feb 15, 1978.) Washington DC: U.S. Government Printing Office, 1978.

Taube, C.A. & Barrett, S.A. (Eds.). *Mental Health, United States, 1983.* (DHHS Publication No. ADM 83-1275). Rockville, MD: National Institute of Mental Health, 1983.

U.S. Department of Health and Human Services, Public Health Service, Division of Nursing. *Source Book—Nursing Personnel.* (DDHS Publication No. HRA 81-21). Washington, DC: U.S. Government Printing Office, 1981.

VandenBos, G.R., Stapp, J., & Kilbury, R.R. Health service providers in psychology: Results of the 1978 APA human resources survey. *American Psychologist* 36(11): 1209, 1981.

Van Stone, W.W. [Survey of chiefs of psychiatry, psychology, social work and psychiatric nursing in a VA psychiatric center regarding role appropriateness of 67 mental health related tasks]. Unpublished study. Palo Alto, CA: Veterans Administration Medical Center, 1978.

2

PROBLEMS IN MENTAL HEALTH CARE

The Untreated Mentally Ill

A critical review of outcome studies of deinstitutionalization points out that its effectiveness depends on the availability of appropriate programs for care in the community (Braun et al., 1981; Pasamanick, 1981). It is clear that many patients discharged from public mental hospitals under the banner of "deinstitutionalization" did not make the transition from inpatient to outpatient care in spite of the near doubling of outpatient activity in the last decade. Furthermore, many may have moved from moderately humane and well-run state hospitals to more primitive community settings where their personal freedom and lifestyle are severely restricted.

Bachrach (1982) notes that many interventions offered in the community to young adult chronic patients are irrelevant to their needs. A good deal of attention is being given to this group (35 and under), which is steadily increasing. Hopper, Baxter, & Cox (1982), considering the same population, deplore bureaucratic policies that segregate responsibility for basic life supports from the responsibility for therapeutic attention. These deficiencies, of course, affect all age groups. Unless the basic needs of food, clothing, shelter, cleanliness, medical care, transportation, and some financial support are available, the patients' ability and motivation to seek and continue psychiatric care are sharply curtailed. For the most part, the mental health and the welfare systems are uncoordinated, to the detriment of these patients.

Many patients are housed in facilities where food and lodging are provided but ongoing psychiatric treatment is not available.

Alternatively, there are board and care homes, as well as skilled nursing facilities, where patients can be held under the aegis of a court-appointed conservator under conditions that may be worse than the level of care seen in even the poorer state hospitals (Lamb, 1979; Lamb 1980).

Surveys of arrest rates of deinstitutionalized patients, as well as the incidence of their detention in jails, have led several authors to describe the "criminalization" of mentally disordered behavior (Lamb & Grant, 1982; Steadman, Cocozza, & Melick, 1978; Steadman, Vanderwyst, & Ribner, 1978). A recent study of 43 jails disclosed that mental health services are being provided by trained workers when they are available (Runck, 1983). Thus, some modicum of organized services is possible even in these restrictive settings, depending on fiscal constraints.

However, for the ambulatory patients some well-intentioned agencies, in fact, provide services that contribute to the neglect of the very patients they are intended to serve. The fact that there are too few agencies, and that these are underfunded, further undermines patient survival. Between 1965 and 1982 the number of hospitalized mental patients in New York State decreased from 80,000 to 23,000 (Hopper, Baxter, & Cox 1982). In 1979 official estimates reported 36,000 homeless people in New York City, either permanently or periodically. At least half of these were mentally disabled, many with a history of psychiatric hospitalization. Public and private shelters at that time could accommodate 4,200 persons ("Another Round," 1982).

Rousseau (1981), in her first-hand study of "shopping bag ladies," describes the multiple determinants of the homelessness of these women. Many have been discharged from state hospitals with nothing except carfare to metropolitan welfare offices and a few days' supply of medication. Often, after years of hospitalization, they lack the social and cultural skills to cope with modern-day living. They are unwanted by family, have no friends and no place to go. If they somehow enter the maze of psychiatric and social agencies, they may be confused by endless forms, conflicting appointment times and lack of any coordinated plan.

Public-assistance agencies may offer housing in rooming houses or single-room occupancy hotels. Problems arising about plumbing, heating, cooking, being robbed or mugged, and other vicissitudes lead some women to seek the safety and independence of the streets—free of agencies, landlords, and other encumbrances. Not infrequently, these women are conspicuously evident sleeping in doorways and under fire escapes during the safer daylight hours. Others sit in railroad or bus stations throughout the day but must not doze, under peril of eviction by the police. They become befogged through sensory deprivation (lack of daylight time and human contact), sleep deprivation, and hunger. Around 11 P.M. many retire to the ladies' room to find shelter for the night, hot water, toilet facilities, and privacy from men. The fortunate ones find an empty booth, shut the door, and stretch out on newspapers for some sleep. However, the police appear to clear them out between 3 and 4 A.M. On departure they leave their "hotel rooms" neat and clean, as evidence of some pride, despite their homeless state.

There are publicly and privately sponsored shelters but not nearly enough to accommodate the thousands seeking a place to sleep. There are many more for men than for women, but most shelters restrict the stay to one or a few nights. Some of these provide good food—hot or cold. Many of the homeless survive on one meal a day. Much of any day may be devoted to finding a meal and a bed.

It is possible to provide better care for deinstitutionalized patients who are homeless? The thousands of needy people involved, the hundreds of agencies that are not coordinated to serve them, and the necessary multimillion-dollar budgets required make the solution of the problem monumental (Goodwin, 1983). The political, economic, social, and humane issues involved are with us every year, particularly during the approach of winter.

One mental health agency in a semirural community reports its involvement in a pilot program that coordinates the fulfillment of the patients' basic needs for food, shelter, clothing, cleanliness, and medical care, as well as provision of psychiatric therapeutic services (W. Klopfenstein, A. Gordon, & D. Carey, personal communication, March, 1983). This approach neutralizes some of the "disjunction between the process of deinstitutionalization and the philosophy that underlies it," as Bachrach (1982, p. 195) has described. In addition, it begins to bridge the gap between the mental health system and the welfare system that was pointed out by Hopper, Baxter, & Cox (1982).

In the last decade the care of many mentally ill patients has shifted from mental health professionals in hospitals to community welfare and voluntary agencies, and to law enforcement personnel. This fact reflects a major quantitative change in the role of all mental health professionals, as well as qualitative changes, in terms of narrowing professional authority and responsibility even when professionals are involved.

Lack of Access by Patients to Effective Treatments

Problems in Organized Care

There are some problems that are inherent in organized psychiatric treatment settings. A previous GAP Report by the Committee on Governmental Agencies (Group for the Advancement of Psychiatry, 1976) carefully analyzed the effects of salaries and other third-party payments on treatment of patients in both private and organized settings. The philosophic and economic thrust of each type of organized setting clearly has a profound effect on the variety, quality, and limits of care. Problems relating to differences between biological, behavioral, social, and psychodynamic viewpoints are still seen in most mental health settings, but are not clearly discipline related. Inadequate funding generally leads to a smaller staff that is less well trained and can do less. The unattractive reputation of many chronic or seriously ill mental patients, often seen in public mental health settings, adds to the general burdens of staff and patients alike in working in or seeking help from bureaucratic institutions. Additional limitations include the relative youth of the mental health sciences and our inability, even in organized settings, to evaluate treatment outcomes well enough to consistently obtain ongoing corrective feedback.

The Mental Health "Team"

There are important problems with the mental health teams seen in most organized settings. In order to function within the "team," the psychiatrist, as well as other members, must become competent in the complexities of leadership and interdisciplinary team management, tasks requiring uncommon skills not significantly related to the training of any mental health practitioner. Furthermore, the benefits of a team of experts with differing skills and backgrounds are diminished when, in fact, they begin to share the same information and perform the same duties. Whether the benefits to patients of input from a multidisciplinary team exceed the considerable cost in extra staffing, training, meeting time, and miscommunications is an open question.

Deprofessionalization of Community Mental Health Centers

A major challenge to traditional roles of all mental health professionals started in the 1960s when ideological arguments for the place of psychosocial factors in the causation of mental illness were first being articulated. Besides the use of teams to maximize integration of the multiple aspects of patient care, community mental health leaders promoted the blurring of role boundaries between individual disciplines, ostensibly allowing one practitioner to maintain continuity of care throughout the system. They also promoted the use of local paraprofessionals, who were assumed to have a greater rapport with indigenous populations and to be more keenly attuned to psychosocial issues in the local community than their more traditionally trained team members (Levenson, 1970). In particular, the increasing use of these relatively untrained paraprofessionals in CMHCs left many of the more highly trained specialists—who had been taught the importance of sophisticated intrapsychic and interpersonal causative factors—convinced that patient care would inevitably suffer. Such a belief extends down the hierarchy, with each discipline becoming concerned, when therapeutic and diagnostic endeavors are placed in the hands of any group with less specialized training.

Psychiatrists are the most adamant in their belief that patient care has suffered. The Task Force on Community Mental Health Centers of the American Psychiatric Association (1972) offered "triage, evaluation, diagnostic formulation, and assignment to appropriate therapeutic modalities" (p. 18) as tasks that should be reserved for the psychiatrist alone. Other opinions have ranged from that of including only diagnosis, drug treatment (Ochberg, 1976), or psychotherapeutic treatment of patients who have associated medical conditions (Mittel, 1978) to direct responsibility for all patient care (Glickman, 1979) as the proper role for psychiatrists. Other mental health professionals strongly disagree with what they perceive as attempts to "turn back the clock."

The burdens that have been shifted from the backs of psychiatrists in these settings do not necessarily fit well on the shoulders of the other core disciplines. The 1969 study of CHMCs by Glasscote and Gudeman (1969) found that 93% of nurses, 78% of social workers, and 48% of psychologists felt inadequately trained for their clinical responsibilities. Thirty-two percent of psychiatrists likewise reported inadequacies in training for treating patients in a CMHC environment.

Problems have been most obvious in CMHCs where the traditional hierarchy has been most seriously challenged by a value system that attempts to make the members of all disciplines egalitarian "generalists." By leveling the traditional hierarchy, CMHC administrators face both the resentment of those whose privileges have been lost as well as the negative feelings of those who perceive residual distinctions (such as salary) as placing them at a relative disadvantage.

Psychiatrists have consistently been found to show the lowest degree of identification with community mental health idealogy (Glasscote & Gudeman, 1969; Robin & Wagenfield, 1977; Winslow, 1978). Their disenchantment with being relegated to an ill-defined supportive role or to the position of monitoring the work of other professionals, in place of the leadership role that they, as physicians, expect themselves to assume, has led many psychiatrists to leave CMHCs. The result of the gradual deprofessionalization seen in CMHCs is that effective treatment for a number of patients, particularly those with significant mental illness, is likely to be unavailable.

Increasing Economic Barriers

Reimbursement Criteria

The rapid inflation of the late 1970s placed an increasing burden on funding of all health care in the United States. In particular, the cost of hospitalization has come under scrutiny. The health insurance industry has traditionally tended to limit psychiatric or other mental health benefits compared to benefits for general medical or surgical treatment, and this tendency has intensified under pressure to economize. The federal government, which has direct control over health care reimbursement in a number of large programs, has an enormous influence over what is done in both public and private sectors.

Medicare. Nationally the over-65 population is the lowest utilizer of mental health services (Goldensohn, 1977). Reimbursement of nonmedical personnel is very limited under Medicare and then may be done only when prescribed by a physician (except for some testing procedures by psychologists). Furthermore, Medicare limits the coverage for psychiatric outpatient treatment in the open market to a maximum per year of $250 or 50% of "reasonable charges," whichever is less, after a $60 deductible is met. Medicare's definition of reasonable charges is uniformly less than the standard in a given community. Inpatient care is limited to 190 days per lifetime for mental health hospitalization. There is no similar ceiling for other medical care. Both of these factors serve to limit mental health treatment of the elderly by all disciplines.

In a further attempt to control the federal health care budget, the Congress, by enacting Public Law 9821 in early 1984, initiated a precedent-shattering prospective payment system in which all Medicare reimbursement to inpatient health care providers would be lump sum based on the primary diagnosis (or procedure) given a patient during each episode of hospital treatment. An elaborate technology using diagnostic related groups (DRGs) was worked out at Yale University and trial tested in New Jersey (Igelhart, 1983). Thus reimbursements from Medicare will be essentially independent of the patient's length of stay and, more importantly, independent of costs to the providers. Because of a relatively small data base regarding psychiatric diagnosis in the New Jersey sample, Congress exempted over 1,500 psychiatric hospitals, psychiatric units in general hospitals, and certain short-term psychiatric hospitals. However, the intent is to include psychiatry in this funding methodology. An analogous system for outpatient reimbursement is also in a developmental stage. The result of this new reimbursement system will be to discourage any but brief hospitalizations in spite of medical need and may sometimes pit treating physicians against hospital administrators with respect to issues of quality of care. Whether the system will actually control costs is still problematic (Wennberg, McPherson, & Caper, 1984).

Medicaid. This program is state administered and thus the regulations vary from state to state. Some states provide direct reimbursement to psychologists and social workers and others do not.

In 1983, in a precedent-setting act, the California state legislature passed Assembly Bill 3480, which authorized Medi-Cal (its Medicaid) *and private insurance carriers* to contract with a limited number of hospitals or other provider groups (such as professional provider organizations [PPOs]) at a prespecified rate. Previously, Medi-Cal paid a portion of the "usual and customary" costs for a given treatment or hospitalization. While this legislation offers a new attempt to control escalating health costs for both the state and private insurance carriers, it poses a serious break with the concepts of one high level of care for rich and poor alike and of freedom of choice for patients. Furthermore, it forces the private practitioner to either join a group or forgo third-party payments. A more serious threat to psychiatrists and their patients is the tendency for some of the PPOs to insist that patients be seen by a primary care doctor before referral to any specialist or to define a patient as "chronic" and exclude him or her from further services after a certain, often minimal, period of treatment. Whether these systems will be found cost-effective is still not settled (Gould, 1984).

CHAMPUS. The Civilian Health and Medical Program for the Uniformed Services and their dependents has traditionally been the most liberal of the federal reimbursement programs with regard to mental health benefits. Many services are covered up to 80%, and psychologists as well as physicians are eligible for direct reimbursement. Social workers may bill through a physician and must work under physician supervision.

Federal employee health benefits. Several of the insurance programs in which federal employees may enroll at one time provided adequate mental health benefits and placed mental health care on a par with physical health care. Escalating overall medical costs led insurers to seek ways to cut benefits, and mental health coverage was the first to be cut. This selective cutback demonstrates the powerlessness of the mental health position in the health field, in spite of evidence supporting the cost-effectiveness of mental health care (Group for the Advancement of Psychiatry, 1976), and may provide a pattern for other insurers.

Budget Limits in Public Mental Health

While some of the mental health budgets in federal, state, county, and city programs may not have actually been cut, the high inflation rate over the last decade has permitted the governing bodies to effectively cut budgets by staying behind inflation. Thus, in spite of a period in the 1960s and early 1970s of unprecedented federal mental health funding, most current governmental programs are feeling the pinch.

Funding for health programs within the Veterans Administration has generally kept pace with inflation. However, in order to maintain credibility with the Congress, the VA is also phasing in the same DRG cost-control technology seen with Medicare in the private sector. The impact on veteran patients with chronic mental illness is unclear at this time, but it would appear that patients requiring more time in treatment than the upper "trim point" will only be reimbursed at 80% of cost.

References

Another Round for the Homeless [Editoral]. *New York Times*, p.28, June 15, 1982.
Bachrach, L.L. Young adult chronic patients: An analytic review of the literature. *Hospital and Community Psychiatry*, 33:189–197, 1982.
Braun, P., Kochansky, G., Shapiro, R., Greenberg, S., Gudeman, J.E., Johnson, S., & Shore, M.F. Overview: deinstitutionalization of psychiatric patients. A Critical Review of Outcome Studies. *American Journal of Psychiatry*, 138:736, June 1981.
Glasscote R.M., & Gudemen, J.E. *The Staff of the Mental Health Center: A Field Study*. Washington, DC: Joint Information Service of the American Psychiatric Association and the National Association for Mental Health, 1969.
Glickman, L: The continuing demedicalization of psychiatry. *Psychiatric Opinion*, 16(5):15–21, 1979.
Goldensohn, S.S. Cost utilization and utilization review of mental health services in a prepaid group practice plan. *American Journal of Psychiatry*, 134(11): 1222–1226, 1977.
Goodwin, M. Cost to shelter homeless in city climbing sharply. *New York Times*, p. 1, October 22, 1983.
Gould, B.S. Why PPOs cannot work. *Northern California Psychiatric Society Newsletter*, p. 2, November 1984.
Group for the Advancement of Psychiatry. Committee on Governmental Agencies. *The Effect of Method of Payment on Mental Health Care. Report No. 95*, New York: Mental Health Materials Center, 1976.
Hopper, K., Baxter, E., & Cox, S. Not making it crazy: The young homeless patients in New York City. In B. Pepper & H. Ryglewicz (Eds.), *The Young Adult Chronic Patient*. San Fransisco: Jossey-Bass, 1982.
Igelhart, J.D. Medicare begins prospective payment of hospitals. *New England Journal of Medicine*, 1428:32, 1983.
Lamb, H.R. The new asylums in the community. *Archives of General Psychiatry*, 36:129, 1979.
Lamb, H.R. Structure: The neglected ingredient of community treatment. *Archives of General Psychiatry*, 37:1224, 1980.
Lamb, H.R. & Grant, R.W. The mentally ill in an urban county jail. *Archives of General Psychiatry*, 39:17, 1982.

Levenson, A.I. Staffing. In N. Grunebaum (Ed.), *The Practice of Community Mental Health.* Boston: 1970. Little, Brown, & Co.

Mittel, N.S. Does the psychiatrist bring anything special to psychotherapy? *Psychiatric Opinion,* 15(4):32–25, 1978.

Ochberg, F.M. Community mental health center legislation: Flight of the Phoenix. *American Journal of Psychiatry,* 133:56–61, 1976.

Pasamanick, B. Deinstitionalization studies: Some clarifications. *American Journal of Psychiatry,* 138:1633, 1981.

Robin, S.S. & Wagenfield, M.O. Psychiatrists in commmunity mental health centers. *Administration in Mental Health,* 4(1):29–41, 1977.

Rousseau, A.M. *Shopping Bag Ladies: Homeless Women Speak About Their Lives.* New York: Pilgrim Press, 1981.

Runck, B. Study of 43 jails shows mental health services and inmate safety are compatible. *Hospital and Community Psychiatry,* 34:1007, 1983.

Steadman, H.J., Cocozza, J.J., & Melick, M.E. Explaining the increased arrest rate among mental patients: The changing clientele of state hospitals. *American Journal of Psychiatry* 135:816, 1978.

Steadman, H.J., Vanderwyst, D., & Ribner, S. Comparing arrest rates of mental patients and criminal offenders. *American Journal of Psychiatry,* 135:1218, 1978.

Task Force Report. *Community Mental Health Centers.* Unpublished report. Washington, DC: American Psychiatric Association, 1972.

Wennberg, J.E., McPherson, K., & Caper, P. Will payments based on diagnostic related groups control hospital costs? *New England Journal of Medicine,* 311:295–300, 1984.

Winslow, W.W. Psychiatric exodus from community mental health centers. *Hospital and Community Psychiatry,* 29:407, 411, 414, 1978.

Section II

THE PROVIDERS

3

PSYCHIATRY: A SPECIALTY OF MEDICINE

Basic Tenets

Psychiatry is that branch of medicine whose members specialize in the treatment of patients with mental disorders. Mental disorders are clinically significant behavioral, cognitive, or emotional syndromes that are associated with a painful symptom or impairment in one or more important areas of functioning. Treatments involve actions to relieve pain and restore functioning. As a medical specialty, psychiatry is distinct from other mental health disciplines in its ability to assume medical responsibility for the mentally ill, to determine the diagnoses in a comprehensive manner, and to implement integrative treatment approaches.

Over the last few years, psychiatric leaders have emphasized psychiatry's basic identity with the field of medicine rather than continuing unfruitful debates over the relative importance of biologic, psychodynamic, or social aspects of the field. Modern medicine itself stresses the reciprocal interaction of mind, body, and society and in that context should be seen as an integrative field rather than identified only with its biological aspects. Since World War II the advances in the understanding of these interactions have allowed the profession to be increasingly helpful to many patients. By defining psychiatric diagnoses on the basis of descriptive criteria, the third edition of the American Psychiatric Association's *Diagnostic and Statistical Manual* (APA, 1980a) improves the reliability of psychiatric diagnosing in the face of increasing complexities in the interaction of biopsychosocial formulations as to the cause of a patient's illness (Leighton, 1982).

Mental disorders fall within the framework of medical illnesses in a number of ways. Most importantly, a growing number of mental disorders, such as the major affective disorders, are associated with demonstrable neurophysiologic and neurochemical changes. A strong genetic component to many of these disorders also emphasizes their similarity to many other medical illnesses. Furthermore, major mental disorders carry a potential for death or disability that is similar to the gravity of other severe medical disorders. We have also known for years that certain mental disorders, such as anorexia nervosa, have profound physical manifestations. Physical illnesses, such as thyroid disease, often have psychiatric manifestations, and, in fact, many traditional medical illnesses, such as peptic ulcer and other "psychosomatic" conditions, are significantly affected by mental components. We acknowledge that, like a number of medical "illnesses," many mental disorders are still incompletely understood so that their classification is based on symptom clusters rather than on etiology.

Training

Basic psychiatric training is achieved through four years of college and four years of medical school, followed by one year of internship and a minimum of three years of psychiatric residency. During the first few years, medical students intensively study basic sciences such as anatomy, bacteriology, biochemistry, genetics, pharmacology, and physiology. Clinical experiences and responsibilities in psychiatry and in the medical and surgical specialities usually begin during the third and fourth years of medical school and progress during internship and the residency training program in emergency rooms, hospitals, and clinic settings. Opportunity for participating in basic and clinical research is available during the entire course of training, and in some settings is required. For psychiatrists, the training progressively emphasizes the biological, psychological, and social aspects of human behavior. The medical identity forged in four years of medical school is solidified by four additional years of residency training. During this process the young psychiatrist develops a crucial sense of medical responsibility for patients' lives and welfare, as well as sensitivity to how patients perceive and organize experience. Together, these qualities affect all aspects of interactions between patients and psychiatrists.

Many psychiatrists seek further specialized training in areas such as psychoanalysis, family therapy, group therapy, or child therapy. These educational programs, often pursued on a part-time basis, entail between one and 10 years of additional continuing study. Since psychiatrists are expected to keep abreast of the field throughout their professional careers, the American Psychiatric Association and many state licensing boards require documented courses in continuing medical education as a condition of continued accreditation.

Sites for Practice

Psychiatrists practice their profession within every health care delivery system. These include private practice, HMOs, CMHCs, student health settings, general hospitals, and specialized psychiatric hospitals, as well as government-funded settings such as county and state hospitals and clinics, Veterans Administration medical centers, and the armed services.

Licensure and Certification

A license to practice medicine issued by state governments is required for the practice of psychiatry. An intensive state or national board examination, covering all aspects of medicine, must be passed to qualify for medical licensure. After four years of postgraduate training, including at least three specifically in psychiatry, the psychiatrist is eligible to be examined by the American Board of Psychiatry and Neurology. The psychiatrist who successfully passes the examination is then certified by the Board as a Diplomate in Psychiatry. The Board has certified approximately 60% of practicing psychiatrists.

Uniqueness and Limitations of Psychiatry

The unique strengths of psychiatry stem from its being a branch of medicine. Primarily, it is the psychiatrist, in contrast to those in the other mental health disciplines, who is held accountable for the evaluation and treatment of anyone with a mental disorder. While specific knowledge has changed over time, psychiatrists have continued to carry this *responsibility*.

Psychiatry, as is true for medicine in general, is *a profession of healing actions*. Clinically, the knowledge and theories that guide these actions are judged on their abilities to help the psychiatrist act effectively. Etiological concepts most useful to physicians are those that offer a variable that the physician can control. For example, physicians knew in the last century that general paresis (resulting from syphilis) could be prevented by controlling indiscriminate sexual behavior. Obviously, however, society did not provide the physician with the authority to prevent such activity. By the first half of this century, paresis had become a major mental disorder responsible for filling thousands of hospital beds in this country. As a result of biological knowledge, physicians were given the ability to destroy the infecting organism by administering penicillin. After this treatment became available in the 1940s, the resulting decrease in paresis was remarkable. Note that while one could "accurately" regard paresis within the context of a social theory, medicine was not helplessly wedded to that theory as the only approach. Medicine is free to search any field of knowledge that may assist its goal as a healing art.

Psychiatry carries with it the impressive *tradition of scientific research* and *achievement* that has characterized medicine throughout this century. In spite of problem areas (see Chapter 2), the care of the great majority of psychiatric patients has vastly improved compared to only 40 years ago and has paralleled, if not exceeded, the success achieved in the rest of medicine. These achievements have come about primarily as a result of a rigorous, international scientific effort supported by private and governmental funding. Psychiatry is unique, in contrast to other mental health disciplines, in synthesizing the medical, psychological, and sociological sciences. Training and experience within this *broad spectrum of scientific knowledge* are the basic strengths of the psychiatrist.

Medicine is an art that searches for *pragmatic solutions;* medicine is not *primarily* a science searching for explanations. The action that a psychiatrist takes in treating a patient may be based on knowledge from one of the sciences, on collective or individual experience, on reason, on intuition, or on some combination of these.

In conceptualizing the practice of healing, we emphasize that the practice of psychiatry, like that of the rest of medicine, is an art that uses the sciences and yet *must frequently extend beyond the knowledge of the sciences.* For centuries societies have placed an enormous value on the health of their members, and physicians have been expected to take actions to address these needs, even in the face of scientific uncertainty. In an initial interview with a patient, for example, the psychiatrist finds that there are hundreds of moments when an action is called for—words, silence, or nonverbal communications, with numerous choices at each point. The specific actions taken may be based upon a theory about human behavior, clinical experience, reason, or intuition, but very few of these actions in an interview are scientifically based. It is impractical to design controlled scientific studies regarding what specific actions should be taken or what statements should be made in the initial interview. The initial interview, nonetheless, is a crucial part of the management of mental disorders. Psychiatry is an art that addresses the total patient.

Unique Skills

An important feature of the healing tradition is the *physician-patient relationship.* This relationship is a special kind of bond characterized by reciprocal trust and respect and by a common goal—the restoration of health. This therapeutic alliance provides a foundation upon which all psychiatric and other medical practice rests and aids healing, whether the interventions be psychodynamic, psychopharmacologic, or psychosocial. Furthermore, a good physician-patient relationship is often vital in obtaining a reliable history of the illness and in performing a competent psychiatric examination.

Another important psychiatric function is *establishing the psychiatric diagnosis.* A psychiatrist is expected to have the skills to obtain the necessary findings and the knowledge to use these findings in order to determine the nature and characteristics of the specific mental disorder. Determining the diagnosis often requires differentiating between a number of possible disorders: for example, ruling out substance abuse disorders before making the diagnosis of a schizophreniform disorder, or ruling out a thyroid disorder before making the diagnosis of an affective disorder. This ruling-out process also requires a broad knowledge of nonpsychiatric medical disorders.

A third important function of psychiatrists is their ability to utilize any or all combinations of the sciences in order to *decide upon the optimum treatment(s)*. The expectation that the psychiatrist will utilize relevant elements of any science encourages an integrative thinking, or "systems approach." Further, in contrast to other clinical disciplines, some of the sciences, such as neurophysiology and neurochemistry, while potentially available conceptually to other disciplines, are available only to physicians for therapeutic action, for example, prescribing medications. Yet the psychiatrist does much more than prescribe medications. The "something extra" that psychiatrists bring to a treatment includes broad, integrative considerations. For example, when confronted with a patient who is receiving a potent antipsychotic medication and who expresses a recent increase in fearfulness, the psychiatrist may need to separate the apprehension associated with the patient's increased awareness of being mentally ill from the restlessness (akathisia) resulting from a side effect of the medication and from the anxiety that is part of the disorder. Only psychiatrists can be held accountable for this multisystem understanding.

In summary, the unique skills of the psychiatric physician include:

1. establishing and maintaining a patient-physician relationship;
2. formulating accurate diagnoses from a comprehensive medical perspective, that is, combining all aspects of biopsychosocial understanding; and
3. utilizing in-depth knowledge of a wide range of sciences in deciding upon the treatment of choice.

Psychiatrists have made great gains since the mid-1940s in their capacity to treat mental disorders, and we believe that further great strides are forthcoming. Yet criticism from a variety of quarters reminds us that psychiatry has not yet found all the answers. From the perspective of those critics preferring a discipline whose body of knowledge is exact, objective, and universally accepted, there are still parts of psychiatry's body of knowledge that may appear disappointingly unclear, subjective, and conflictual. From the perspective of those wanting answers to the age-old questions of what is the "mind," what is the answer to the nature-nurture dispute, or similar issues, psychiatry has no pat answers. For those critics preferring a discipline that remains totally within a single scientific framework, psychiatry does not meet this expectation inasmuch as it uses many theories and sciences. Those desiring a diagnostic system that ties a specific diagnosis to etiology or to a specific treatment may be dissatisfied that some psychiatric diagnoses are still aggregations of syndromes that are not directly related to etiology or to treatment. These issues point out the limitations in psychiatry's knowledge base; but if the field limited itself to proven facts, or to "mind" to the exclusion of "brain," to one scientific framework, or to treatment of patients with fully understood diagnoses, it would be moving away from its healing role. While we continue to desire clarity, exactness, and final answers, gains in these directions must be achieved without the healers losing their effectiveness with their patients.

Over the past three decades, the ability of psychiatrists to treat patients with mental disorders has been enhanced by psychotherapeutic approaches, including psychoanalytic, cognitive, behavioral, family and learning theory models; by pharmacological advances, including medications that are increasingly effective for certain syndromes; as well as by the milieu and system constructs characteristic of social approaches. Since psychiatry draws upon these diverse areas of knowledge, another sort of criticism of psychiatry arises from this very diversity. In particular, professionals who are primarily oriented to psychology, to biology, or to one of the social sciences perceive the other two areas as absorbing too much of psychiatry's focus and missing what psychiatry has "most to offer." While it has been somewhat easier to use the scientific method to resolve both theoretical and therapeutic differences within the psychopharmacological perspective, this methodology remains relatively unsophisticated with regard to resolving conflicts among or between psychologically and socially oriented professionals.

Despite the complaints about psychiatric knowledge, *the diversity of psychiatry* provides a flexibility for integrating elements from many fields that can well serve our patients. Psychiatry benefits many patients whose illnesses and the consequences of these illnesses are not fully addressed within another specialty's therapeutic range. The so-called "problem patients" of medicine, surgery, and pediatrics need the integrative conceptualization that psychiatrists can often provide. For example, consultation and liaison provided by psychiatrists in general medical hospitals have proven clinically and economically useful (see p. 103–109). Thus, while some find the ferment of psychiatry disquieting, in actuality this diversity also represents a strength. Today's psychiatrist integrates psychological, milieu, family, and physiological aspects in the evaluation and treatment of patients with complicated illnesses.

In Chapter 6 we address the *exploding knowledge base* of psychiatry over the last few decades. This recent expansion of knowledge, however, has made the task of remaining current in all aspects of the treatment of the mentally ill increasingly difficult for psychiatrists and has led many to specialize. Specialization in one area of psychiatry, however, tends to narrow the psychiatrist's perspective. By specializing in only one form of therapy, for example, some psychiatrists may have lost the capacity *to fully evaluate* a new patient. The profession must address the role of the highly specialized psychiatrist when that specialization is associated with a loss of ability to provide comprehensive evaluations of mentally ill patients.

Both funding agencies and the general public express concern that the cost of *treatment by psychiatrists is more expensive* than the cost of treatment by "other mental health disciplines." These concerns seem especially true if considering only a specific task, such as a session of individual psychotherapy. (Although in many areas of the country, clinical psychologists charge essentially the same as

psychiatrists for individual psychotherapy.) Important, but difficult to measure, is the cost versus the potential benefit in terms of
treating the whole illness, as opposed to the cost of a single service.
It is our belief that psychiatrists offer a service that is fundamen-
tally different from that of other mental health professionals. The
complexity of mental disorders with their often interacting genetic-
organic, emotional, cognitive, and social components, demands a
diagnostician/therapist well versed in all of these areas. Such ills are
generally not static, unchanging symptom complexes that vary only
in degree as the condition's severity grows or responds to treatment.
Major depression and the psychoses, as well as a host of less severe
afflictions, often display a complex evolution of interplay between
their constituent biopsychosocial factors, which require frequent
reassessment and reformulation of treatment strategy. Only psychiatric training, with its emphasis on the synthesis of these areas into
comprehensive and ongoing diagnostic formulations, provides an
adequate background.

   We must also consider the additional benefits that a psychiatrist
brings to these tasks in terms of not only basic knowledge and skills,
but also the positive effects of a medical authority and responsibility and the ability to provide a comprehensive, ongoing evaluation. In psychotherapy, psychiatrists are accountable for the breadth
of mental illness, accountable to do therapeutic work in depth,
with all components of the mind, and to understand and treat
as needed the many influences of biological, neurological, and
hormonal or biochemical connections and interactions. *Psychotherapy by psychiatrists* includes the special ability to recognize, diagnose, and treat, with a variety of somatic and pharmacologic means,
the various crises as they occur during psychotherapy. Medical
training gives the psychiatrist a special ability to recognize and
differentiate changing states and degrees of morbidity that occur
during a course of treatment and to intervene with special medical
treatments, security measures, or other interventions, as appropriate. The complex process of careful diagnostic assessment and
of comprehensive treatment planning continues, then, throughout
the course of psychotherapy.

   Some of the economic concerns about the costs of psychiatric treatment will be alleviated when we have more clearly defined the differences between illness and problems in living. Furthermore, misconceptions about the true cost of psychiatric treatment will be allayed when we achieve greater clarity with regard to indications for psychotherapy, as opposed to counseling or to an educational approach.

A remaining concern of psychiatry is its possible *misuse to oppress people* on the basis of race, gender, ethnic background, class, political actions, or deviant behavior. Unfortunately, adherence to the Hippocratic tradition, while helpful, is no guarantee that the healers will be immune from the prejudices of the society to which they belong. Thus, psychiatrists must be vigilant to avoid misusing their power.

Economics

Psychiatrists' earnings are less than most other medical specialists, averaging about $70,000 a year in 1980. The personal cost of becoming a psychiatrist is now approaching $100,000 for college and medical school. Additionally, some psychiatrists undergo a personal psychoanalysis or other training program as part of their postgraduate training that costs them additionally many thousands of dollars.

Relationships with Other Disciplines
(Joint Commission, 1986)

Psychiatrists and other mental health professionals are generally trained, among other skills, to perform psychotherapy, broadly defined. The other disciplines are licensed to perform psychotherapy within their own areas of uniqueness and expertise. They are taught to be alert to signs and symptoms that suggest a mental illness but are not expert in diagnosing or treating the specific illness. For that, they must refer to the physician—the psychiatrist.

A large mental health system may employ 50 or more different disciplines that contribute to the care of the mentally ill. Moreover, many patients obtain important support from families, communities, and churches with whom clinicians must be in touch. As the number and roles of various disciplines have increased, both in and out of institutions, so have the needs for guidelines regarding professional relationships between the disciplines. Generally, the psychiatrist relates with others serving the mentally ill in one of four clinical types of relationships:* 1) supervisory; 2) collaborative; 3) consultative; and 4) independent referral.

A *supervisory relationship* is an ongoing one in which the psychiatrist provides professional directions and active guidance to working with patients. The psychiatrist is responsible for the initial evaluation, diagnosis, and prescription of a treatment plan. The psychiatrist remains responsible for the patient's treatment as long as the treatment continues under supervision (APA, 1980b).

In the *collaborative relationship* both participants share a negotiated responsibility for the patient's treatment, in accordance with the qualifications and limitations of each discipline's abilities. The patient must be informed of each discipline's respective responsibility in the patient's treatment. The psychiatrist is responsible for periodic evaluations of the patient's status, to be certain that collaboration continues to be appropriate. Here, each collaborating discipline is serving the patient independently (APA, 1980b).

In the *consultative relationship* the psychiatrist does not assume responsibility for the patient's treatment. The relationship is initiated by another physician or by another discipline. The psychiatrist evaluates the patient or evaluates information provided by another discipline and offers a psychiatric opinion that the other discipline may or may not use.

APA guidelines state that psychiatrists should not continue to supervise, collaborate, or consult if they ascertain that their roles are being misrepresented or if convinced that the care being provided is either inappropriate or inadequate. An exception may be when the psychiatrist specifically accepts a responsibility with the goal of improving the quality of care so that the care will become adequate. Psychiatrists with an ongoing supervisory or collaborative relationship should maintain such relationships with

---

*We are not addressing administrative relationships.

other disciplines only if they are able to keep appropriately informed about the nature of the treatment and the progress of their patients. They must feel assured that the treatment provided by the nonphysician practitioner is being carried out competently and adequately. This constraint may require the psychiatrist to personally examine the patient from time to time. The basic tenet of these interdisciplinary relationships is that the patient must benefit (APA, 1980b).

A fourth type of clinical relationship is an *independent referral* by a psychiatrist to another physician or to a member of a nonmedical discipline.* Some examples of referrals by a psychiatrist might include an alcohol-dependent person being referred to Alcoholics Anonymous; a patient with a stuttering problem being referred to a speech therapist; a patient with primary degenerative dementia from a remote rural setting being referred to a visiting psychiatric nurse for counseling and follow-up evaluations; or a couple with a marital problem being referred to a psychiatric social worker for marriage or family counseling. In independent referrals psychiatrists terminate their responsibility for the patient. They believe that the patient's interest is well served by this referral.

In order to provide a broad base of mental health care and treatment, especially when working with severely, chronically ill patients, care and treatment from a number of disciplines should be encouraged. Therefore, it is important for the psychiatrist to achieve effective working relationships with colleagues from other disciplines in order to provide the optimal level of psychiatric care and treatment for such patients.

We now refer the reader interested in other disciplines to the Appendices, which describe clinical psychologists (Appendix A), clinical social workers (Appendix B), and psychiatric/mental health nurses (Appendix C). These chapters represent the views of their authors and have not been edited by GAP members. Indeed, we discuss our disagreements with many of their opinions in Chapter 5.

---

*Unlike the other three types of relationships, the American Psychiatric Association has no guideline on the practice of independent referral.

References

American Psychiatric Association. *Diagnostic and Statistical Manual of Mental Disorders (3rd ed.).* Washington, DC: Author, 1980a.

American Psychiatric Association. Guidelines for psychiatrists in consultative, supervisory, or collaborative relationships with non-medical therapists. *American Journal of Psychiatry,* 137:1489–1491, 1980b.

Joint Commission on Interprofessional Affairs. *Guidelines for Interprofessional Relationships in the Mental Health Field.* Unpublished document, 1986. (Available from Office of Psychiatric services, American Psychiatric Association, 1400 K St. N.W., Washington, DC, 20005)

Leighton, A.H. *Caring for Mentally Ill People* (p. 221). New York: Cambridge University Press, 1982.

4

PRIMARY CARE: THE LARGEST MENTAL HEALTH DELIVERY SYSTEM

Any assessment of future roles for psychiatry and relationships among the mental health disciplines would be incomplete without consideration of the contribution made by nonpsychiatric physicians working within the primary medical care delivery system. The crucial importance of the primary care physician to the provision of mental health services is emphasized by two facts: 1) primary care physicians treat more patients with diagnosed mental disorders than do all the traditional mental health disciplines combined (Shortell & Daniels, 1974; Rieger, Goldberg, & Taube, 1978); and 2) the majority of persons seeking entry into the primary care system are without evidence of organic pathology and have positive evidence for the existence of psychological factors underlying their symptoms (Engel, 1977; Stoeckle, Zola, & Davidson, 1964; Stoudemire, Thompson, Mitchell, & Grant, 1982–1983).

Epidemiology

The first consideration was recently addressed by Regier and associates (1978) at the National Institute of Mental Health. In their epidemiological study. "The De Facto U.S. Mental Health Services System," these investigators offered documentary evidence that 60% of the estimated 32,000,000 sufferers from mental illness in the United States receive treatment within the primary care system exclusively, with a smaller number (about 6%) being seen in overlap with the specialty mental health sector. These figures contrast with the 21% treated entirely by mental health specialists. Thus only one out of five patients with mental illness, diagnosed as such, is treated by a member of the core mental health disciplines. Primary care physicians treat three out of five, and one in five patients does not receive any specific treatment focused on his or her mental disturbance. A recent study of child patients in Monroe County, New York, found that mental health problems among this population were treated five times more often by pediatricians, than by either an inpatient or outpatient psychiatric facility (Goldberg, Regier, McInenny, Pless, & Roghmann, 1979). The primary care physician is also extensively involved in not only the treatment and follow-up of the mentally ill, but in the initial workup and "labeling" of these patients. Four percent of patient visits to general practitioners, 5% to pediatricians, and 9% to internists lead to a diagnosis of mental illness.

Settings

The extent of the primary care system's contribution to the provision of mental health services is supported by a review of the settings in which patients receive treatment. Hankin and Oktay (1979) report that 43% of the mentally ill are seen in general medical settings, with another 10% treated in general hospitals. This compares with 8% who are treated in community mental health centers, 5% treated in private practice by psychiatrists or psychologists, and 11% treated in mental hospitals, either public or private.

Since less than 8% of the physicians in this country are psychiatrists (Hankin & Oktay, 1979), it is not surprising that a significant percentage of this patient load would come to the attention of the 52% of physicians who practice within a primary care model (Coleman & Patrick, 1976). A 1978 survey of physicians' distribution in the United States (Wanderman, 1979) found that there were 375,811 active physicians in this country, of which 342,714 were involved in patient care. In the primary care specialties, there were 56,197 general and family practitioners, 79,068 internists, 25,570 pediatricians and, as some authors consider them a primary care group for women, 23,963 gynecologists. At the same time, there were 28,522 psychiatrists.

Geographic Distribution

Of the 342, 714 patient care physicians, 87% work in 300 metropolitan areas in which 75% of the population resides (Wanderman, 1979). While the fact that 4.5% of U.S. counties have no physicians is often cited as a proof of physician maldistribution, these areas contain only 0.2% of the population, with an average density of four persons per square mile. Thus, there is currently approximately one primary care physician for every 1,000 U.S. residents, with a fairly even urban/rural distribution. The previously cited preponderance of physicians in metropolitan areas is largely accounted for by the urban concentration of nonprimary care specialists.

Use of Medical Services

Mentally ill persons are high utilizers of medical services and facilities and thus would have considerable contact with the primary care sector, even if they had all their psychiatric care under other auspices. For example, Coleman and Patrick (1978) found that the 16% of patients in an HMO with diagnosed mental illness accounted for 28% of all patient visits to that facility. Other studies have shown that patients with mental illness visit health facilities three to four times as often as patients without mental illness, they require more time per visit (Haupt, Orleans, George, & Brodie, 1980), and their utilization rate remains double the average after their visits for mental health services are excluded.

Undiagnosed Illness

Perhaps the greatest contribution of primary care physicians to mental health lies in their treatment of patients with psychological distress who are neither formally diagnosed as having a psychiatric disorder, nor prone to conceptualizing their help-seeking in psychological terms. Kaufman and Bernstein (1957) reported a poor correlation between identifiable disease and perceived illness in the setting of a general medicine clinic. They studied 1,000 consecutive patients in an ambulatory clinic and found that 69% had no demonstrable organic lesion. The implication is that the majority of patients who identify themselves as ill to a primary care physician have emotional distress related to their presenting complaints. A study by Lipowski (1967) demonstrated this to be the case in 30%–60% of general medicine inpatients and 50%–80% of outpatients, while Kaufman and Bernstein (1957) had such factors identified in 81% of their cohorts. Similar studies conducted by Stoeckle et al. (1964) in the Massachusetts General Hospital medical outpatient clinics showed that 79%–82% of the men and 87%–88% of the women patients revealed psychological distress.

Special Role of the Primary Care Sector in Treatment of Mental Illness

The large numbers of psychologically distressed and mentally ill patients cared for within the primary care sector are not the result of a shortage of mental health specialists alone. Rather, there is good evidence that both the primary care physicians and their patients see the rendering of such care as well within, if not integral to, the primary care physician's expertise. An earlier GAP Report documents that patients expect their physicians to meet their emotional needs (Group for the Advancement of Psychiatry, 1964). In one study, 41% of all visits made to the primary care physician involved the patient's raising some question not specifically related to his physical condition about which he wanted advice (Brown, Robertson, Kosa, & Alpert, 1971). Another study showed that 88% of patients who were fearing an impending "nervous breakdown" chose the primary physician as the first source of help (Enelow, 1966), and still another study found that 74% of the members of the United Auto Workers' Union believed that they could receive appropriate mental health care from their family physicians (Glasser,

Duggan, & Hoffman, 1975). Since 84% of primary care physicians felt "strongly" that they should be involved in the emotional problems of their patients (Harr, Green, Hyamz, & Jaffee, 1972), it is not surprising that most of the cases presenting to primary care physicians are subsequently managed within their practice. Eastwood (1971) reports that only about 10% of the patients that were specifically diagnosed as having emotional problems were referred to a psychiatrist. The referral rate to the specialty mental health sector of less than 1% of all primary care patients prevails across primary care disciplines (Goldberg et al., 1979; Haupt et al., 1980; Locke, Krantz, & Kramer, 1966, Shortell & Daniels, 1974).

Diagnostic Categories Treated by Primary Care

Reviews of the distribution of diagnostic categories of mental illness treated in the primary care setting showed that between 14%–21% of the patients diagnosed as mentally ill are psychotic; 40%–55% are neurotic; 11%–28% have personality disorders; 11% have transient situational disturbances; and 2%–13% have other disorders, including organic brain syndromes (Goldberg, Krantz, & Locke, 1970; Rosen, Locke, Goldberg, & Babigian, 1972). Cutting across these categories, depression was found to be the most commonly designated psychiatric problem treated in the primary care setting (Davies, 1964; Katon, Williamson, & Ries, 1981; Zung, MaGill, Moore, & George, 1983). The most commonly reported problems among the 5% of pediatric patients who were diagnosed as having behavioral disturbances were adaptation reactions (22%); hyperkinetic disorders (19%); psychosomatic disorders (13%); and conduct disorders (13%) (Goldberg et al., 1979). In general, the primary care physician saw fewer phobic, paranoid, severely deteriorated schizophrenic and alcoholic patients than did mental health specialists, but more commonly encountered anxiety, hypochondriasis, and depression (Cooper, 1974). Many mentally ill patients who saw primary care physicians were especially difficult to treat, because they so often presented with ill-defined but tenaciously defended somatic complaints and, unlike the neurotic patients who sought care from the mental health sector, had not accepted their illness in psychological terms (Goldberg & Blackwell, 1970; Kessel, 1965; Rosen, Kleinman, & Katon, 1982).

Effectiveness

Despite this extensive involvement of primary care physicians in the treatment of the mentally ill and the provision of mental health services to the general public, there have been few studies that have systematically examined what diagnostic and treatment procedures these providers use or how effectively they use them. Preliminary research in this area by the biometry branch of the National Institute of Mental Health indicates that primary care physicians self-report the use of some type of supportive "talking" therapy in 84% of the cases of mental disorders coming to their attention, medication in 60%, and the suggestion of specific environmental change in 19% (Rosen et al., 1972). In only 14% of cases did the primary care physicians see themselves using medication as the sole treatment modality.

Unfortunately, an even larger body of research data indicate that one of the major deficiencies in the primary care model for the delivery of mental health services is that the primary care physicians tend to favor a single treatment modality for all patients (Aldrich, 1965). This tendency is apparently related both to general practitioners' needs for treatment strategies that do not require a large commitment of time—the average primary-care physician has 158 patient visits a week—and to limitations in their repertoire of mental health skills (Cassata & Kirkman-Liff, 1981). Although psychiatrists are likely to employ psychotherapy in 91% of all patient visits and drug therapy in only 30%, other medical specialists use psychotherapy in only 22% of visits with patients who have a diagnosis of mental illness, but drug therapy in 67% of such visits (Brown, Regier, & Bolten, 1977; Coleman & Patrick, 1976). These figures, based on outside analysis of what the primary care physicians were doing, are markedly at variance with the previously reported figures of what the primary care physicians were themselves reporting as their treatment modality usage. Thus, although primary physicians reported that they use drug therapy alone in only 14% of cases that involved emotional problems, a combined chart review and interview survey by Fink and Shapiro (1966) disclosed that drugs constituted the only treatment used for over one-half of such patients in primary care settings.

The most common forms of psychiatric treatment used by pediatricians for their emotionally disturbed patients were supportive therapy (86%); suggestions about environmental change (43%); and drugs (16%) (Goldberg et al., 1979). Referral for psychiatric care or consultation was made in 37% of the pediatric cases in which there was psychological impairment, this rate being more than three times that seen for adult patients.

The Advantages of the Primary Care Delivery System

The advantages of the primary care systems in the delivery of mental health services are inherent in the very definition of primary care. Although its essential features may be described somewhat differently by various writers, the elements discussed by Parker (1974) or Alpert and Charney (1974) are representative:

1. It is "first contact" medicine, providing entry, screening, and triage for the rest of the health care system.
2. It assumes "longitudinal responsibility" for the patient in health and disease. Thus it must provide a full range of basic services designed to meet the needs of primary, secondary, and tertiary prevention, as well as care for the common illnesses and disabilities of the target population. It must also ensure access to the services provided.
3. It serves as the "integrationist" for the patient, ensuring the smooth coordination of services throughout the entire process, and eliminating as much delay and duplication as possible.
4. It provides "stabilizing human support" for patients and their families during periods of crisis.

This description, of course, represents an ideal frequently not achieved. As pointed out by several reviewers, *the primary care model delivery system in the United States is, in reality, a nonsystem* (Hankin & Oktay, 1979). Unlike the British National Health Service and other European systems, the entry point for health care in the United States is not uniformly through the primary-care system. Nonetheless, fragmented though it may be, this sector remains the system of care that is most accessible and most frequently used by the U.S. population.

Within the limitations suggested above, the potential advantages of the primary care system with regard to treatment of emotional illness, as outlined by the World Health Organization (1973), are the following:

> Most disturbed patients present physical symptoms and do not identify themselves as needing psychiatric care. Most patients who do recognize the psychological component of their illness do not see themselves as being "sick enough" to entertain a referral for long-term referred psychotherapy, but they often will accept and benefit from short-term intervention, especially for bereavement and anniversary problems (Temperling, 1978).
>
> Psychological and physical illnesses tend to coexist in many patients and may be difficult to separate in diagnosis and treatment. Although the reasons for such coexistence are still not clear, the evidence that patients with emotional disorders suffer from a higher incidence of objectively confirmed physical diseases, than do patients without emotional problems, is substantial and convincing (Ananth, 1984; Eastwood, 1975; Eastwood & Trevalyan, 1972; Hall, Gardner, Popkins, LeCann, & Stickney, 1981; Roessler & Greenfield, 1961; Shepherd, 1973).
>
> A visit to a nonpsychiatric physician involves less stigma than a visit to a psychiatrist. A multitude of studies have reaffirmed this point (Coleman & Patrick, 1976; Morrill, 1978).
>
> A patient under the care of a primary care practitioner is less likely to drift from specialist to specialist than is one without a primary care physician relationship.
>
> Since many psychiatric disorders are related to family prob-

lems, the family practitioner is in an ideal position to provide comprehensive treatment. Many psychiatric patients require long-term follow-up, and the primary care model of brief contacts over extended periods, as opposed to the mental health model of intensive contact over relatively short periods, may enable the primary care physician to be in a preferable position to provide such care.

Several additional advantages based on research within the U.S. health care system may be added to the World Health Organization's list:

The mental health care provided by the primary sector is accessible to specific high-risk populations that are underrepresented in the specialty mental health sector, especially children and the aged (Borus, 1967; Glasser et al., 1975; Tischler, Henisz, Myers, & Buswell, 1975).

Early detection and early treatment (or referral) can improve prospects for preventing some mental illnesses (Morrill, 1978). Locke and Gardner (1969) emphasize that the longer a patient interacts in the same setting, the greater the chance that the staff will correctly label the patient's mental illness. They attribute this increased case finding to three factors: the providers are better able to detect emotional illness within the context of a developing relationship; repeated visits by the patient may raise the suspicion of emotional factors; and patients with a purely physical disorder tend to terminate routine care earlier, leaving a greater proportion of persons with emotional disorders under care.

The treatment of emotional problems within the primary care setting reduces the attrition expected in referral. It also obviates feelings of rejection and abandonment that these patients may experience, in spite of the most skillful referral preparation. Only 10% of patients referred for the first time to a community mental health center and 42% of those re-referred to one, accepted the referral (France, Waddington, & Haupt, 1978). Referral acceptance rates are somewhat higher if made to a specific practitioner, especially if that individual works within the primary care setting (Borus, 1967; Coleman &

Patrick, 1976). Interestingly, 80% of those patients seen for an inpatient psychiatric consultation who were given the choice of being followed after their discharge, either by their primary care physician or at a CMHC, chose the primary care physician. Finally, in a study of patients already on an inpatient psychiatric unit, almost half wanted their family practitioners involved in their aftercare (Lerner & Blackwell, 1975).

The Disadvantages of the Primary Care Delivery System

Despite this extensive involvement of primary care physicians in the treatment of the mentally ill and in the provision of mental health services, there are several major deficiencies in the primary care model of mental health service delivery.

The *first* deficiency is that primary care physicians, as a group, tend to lack sensitivity in the diagnosis of mental illness (Hankin & Oktay, 1979). For example, Eastwood (1971) reported that the psychiatric conditions of 19% of women and 27% of men went undetected within the general practice setting, and Goldberg and Blackwell (1970) showed that one-third of such patients were misdiagnosed. Likewise, Regier and associates (1978) calculated that, although 4% of primary practice patients receive a formal psychiatric diagnosis, 15% probably have diagnosable psychiatric illness.

The reported rate of appropriately diagnosed mental illness tends to be somewhat higher in practices where the primary care physician has had some training in or exposure to psychiatry. For example, in a study that compared the rate of verified psychiatric diagnoses made in a university facility that emphasized the importance of emotional problems with those arrived at in a nonuniversity hospital with a similar patient population, emotional problems were uncovered in 27% of the cases seen in the former setting, but in only 10% in the latter (Rosen et al., 1972).

On the other hand, in a study (Eastwood & Trevalyan, 1972) in which the general practitioner was also trained as a psychiatrist, the emotional problems of one-third of the patients were missed. These patients within the "hidden psychiatric morbidity" group were found to formulate their problems in somatic terms, not only to their doctor, but also to themselves. This study indicates that a significant proportion of the missed psychiatric morbidity in the primary care setting is related to factors that are difficult for even the most knowledgeable or interested physician to control.

The *second* disadvantage to be noted is the finding that the primary care physician frequently lacks a basic philosophy or rationale for intervention with psychotropic medications. Recent studies demonstrated that 31% of the population uses some psychotropic drug each year (Parry, Balter, Mellinger, Cisin, & Manheimer, 1973) and that 14% are on a sedative-hypnotic (Balter, Levine, & Manheimer, 1974). Furthermore, 25% of all patients receiving any type of medication from their physician are receiving a psychotropic drug (Patrick, Eagle, & Coleman, 1978). The problem is compounded for patients with mental illness, since they typically receive three times as many prescriptions as do the nonmentally ill (Coleman & Patrick, 1978; Parry et al., 1973). General practitioners and internists account for the majority of this prescribing; psychiatrists and neurologists are responsible for only about one-third of written prescriptions for psychotropic drugs (Balter & Levine, 1969; Solow, 1975). In fact, 85% of patients using psychotropic drugs have never seen a psychiatrist (Parry et al., 1973).

The problem of the overprescription of psychiatric drugs by the primary care physician is complicated by indications that such drugs are often given to the wrong patients in the wrong doses. One explanation for this, as noted by Balter and Levine (1969), is that primary physicians are more likely to prescribe an agent on the basis of desired action rather than diagnosis. Indeed, several papers (Balter & Levine, 1969; Blackwell, 1973; Parry et al., 1973; Solow, 1975) have indicated that less than half of the patients who receive psychoactive drugs have ever been formally diagnosed as having an emotional illness. While at least some of the psychoactive drugs being given are purportedly being used as adjuvants in the maintenance therapy of common physical problems, the rationale for such usage is, with several notable exceptions, not supported in the literature by well-controlled studies (Cooperstock, 1974). Finally, even in those cases where the appropriate drug for an appropriate patient is being used, primary care physicians all too often prescribe at below therapeutic dosages for fear of potential side effects (Wylon & Weiner, 1967).

A *third* deficiency that arises in considering mental health services provided by the primary care physician is that a significant proportion of primary care physicians simply refuse to treat any psychiatric illness at all or avoid specific categories of emotional disorders. Such refusal may be grounded in the primary care physician's personality, feelings of inadequacy, or biases about patients who have particular behavioral problems. Thus, of those patients who are appropriately diagnosed as being mentally ill by the primary care sector, only 67% receive some form of treatment within that sector, while 5% are referred, leaving 28% who receive no treatment of any kind (Shepherd, Cooper, Brown, & Kalton, 1966). Although primary care physicians are more apt to treat an emotionally ill patient if they have known both the patient and family for years, they are reluctant to treat the chronic psychotic patient or those with problems related to the abuse of drugs or alcohol (Fink, Goldensohn, Shapiro, & Daily, 1967; Hull, 1979; Robertson, 1979; Shepherd et al., 1966; Stanford, 1972).

A *fourth* deficiency exists in the referral relationship between the primary care and specialty mental health sector. The percentage of patients referred depends on various factors, several of which reflect characteristics of the referring physician. For example, referral rates tend to be higher when the primary care physician has a personal interest in psychiatry (Shortell & Daniels, 1974). They also increase in proportion to the physician's age and length of time in practice (Gardner, Peterson, & Hall, 1974). Likewise, the amount of postgraduate training the physician has had is also positively correlated. Shortell and Daniels (1974) found that nearly 11% of the referrals by board-certified internists are made to psychiatrists versus 6%-8% for those not board certified. Of particular interest is the finding in one survey of 1,156 primary physicians (Harr et al., 1972) that those who felt most competent in the handling of psychiatric problems also felt the greatest need for assistance in their care of such patients. Obviously, the availability of mental health specialists is also a variable in determining the rate of referral. For example, in the two-year period after a prepaid group practice setting introduced on-site mental health services, the rate of referrals increased from 6.6 per 1,000 to 11 per 1,000 (Fink et al, 1969).

A number of interesting studies have investigated the motivating factors behind psychiatric referrals from the primary care sector. The consensus of these investigations is that those patients referred were most likely to be young, male, single, and from a low socioeconomic background, compared with the relevant base populations (Gardner et al, 1974; Hopkins & Cooper, 1969; Weiss, Freeborn, & Lamb, 1973). They were also more likely to have chronic, rather than acute, conditions that their physicians considered severe, which interfered markedly with the conduct of their lives, seemed due to life stress, rather than being secondary to medical illness, and seemed likely to benefit from psychiatric treatment, but had not improved under the treatment regimen of the primary care physician (Fink et al., 1967; Fink & Shapiro, 1966). Thus the problems of depression, psychosis, and suicide are especially common reasons for referral (Raft, 1973; Shepherd et al., 1966; Shortell & Daniels, 1974).

Kaesar and Cooper (1971) uncovered a somewhat darker side of the referral process. They found that the reason for referral was frequently based on the primary care physicians' desire to have the mental health system assume clinical responsibility for the patient rather than their desire for consultative advice. Thus, most patients were referred not on the basis of diagnosis, but for abnormalities of conduct, social problems, or "inappropriate responses to medical attention." This tendency led Hankin and Oktay (1979) to conclude, "It is unclear to what extent physicians refer those patients who would most benefit from psychiatric service and to what extent they refer those who have become troublesome to them" (p. 320).

The alienation between psychiatry and other medical specialties (Hankin & Oktay, 1979; Raft, 1973) and the reluctance of many primary-care physicians to "insult" their patients by suggesting psychiatric referral lead to the interesting paradox found in one study (Fink, Shapiro, & Goldensohn, 1970), in which 45% of the patients seen in consultation by psychiatrists had a psychiatric consultation in mind before visiting their primary physician. This group of "self-initiated" referrals were found to be generally better educated, acquainted with mental health resources from past experience, and favorably impressed with psychiatry.

The poor completion of suggested referrals to a mental health specialist may be due in part to the patient's reluctance to lose his relationship with his primary physician. Although 75% of the patients studied found a psychiatric consultation to have been a positive experience while hospitalized on a medical or surgical ward, only 20% were positive about referral to a CMHC, with 80% wanting their primary care physician to manage their follow-up care (France et al., 1978). Furthermore, the "no-show" rate for referral to a mental health specialist decreased from 75% to 23% in a study where the specialist moved into the physical setting of the primary care provider (Morrill, 1978).

Such data as these, then, appear to support the findings of Raft (1973) and Smith (1957) that the major reasons for patients' resisting psychiatric referral have to do with the following: psychiatry's marginal status in the field of medicine, which is all too often communicated to the patient; the patient's fear of emotional illness; and the physician's feelings of frustration and disappointment at being unable to find organic disease. These factors contribute to the patient's feelings of being rejected when referral is made. It is surprising to note, in one study, that neither fear that "talking will do no good," that such referral would prejudice one's job, nor that the cost of psychiatric services might be excessive seem to be significant impediments to the patient's accepting referral (Glasser et al., 1975).

Finally, perhaps the most basic disadvantage of the primary-care model of mental health service delivery is the primary-care physicians' difficulty in handling their patients' defenses of denial, displacement, or hypochondriasis. Because of societal expectations, as well as their own, regarding the role of the "doctor," primary physicians frequently have difficulty confronting the patient with these issues and refraining from the use of symptomatic somatic therapy for the patient's displaced complaints. Thus, the primary care physician must resist powerful internal and outside influences that are aligned with the patient's demand for interventions that the physician may know intellectually to be countertherapeutic (Shemo, 1984). Despite the limitations noted, the primary medical care system remains an extensive, trusted, and valuable component of the mental health delivery.

References

Aldrich C. The general practitioner's approach to emotional problems: A comparative study in two countries. *American Journal of Psychiatry,* 122:504–508, 1965.

Alpert, J., & Charney, E. *The Education of Physicians for Primary Care.* (DHEW Publication No. HRA 74-3113). Washington, DC: U.S. Government Printing Office, 1974.

Ananth, J. Physical illness and psychiatric disorders. *Comprehensive Psychiatry,* 25:586–593, 1984.

Balter, M., Levine, J., & Manheimer, D. Cross-national study of the extent of anti-anxiety/sedative drug use. *New England Journal of Medicine,* 290:769–774, 1974.

Balter, M., & Levine, J. The nature and extent of psychotropic drug usage in the United States. *Psychopharmacological Bulletin,* 4:3–13, 1969.

Blackwell, B. Psychotropic drugs in use today: The role of diazepam in medical practice. *Journal of the American Medical Association,* 225:1637–1641, 1973.

Borus, J. Neighborhood health centers as providers of primary mental health care. *New England Journal of Medicine* 295:140–145, 1967.

Brown, B., Regier, D., & Bolten, M. Key interactions among psychiatric disorders, primary care and the use of psychiatric drugs. *Clinical Anxiety/Tension in Primary Medicine.* Symposium sponsored by The Excerpta Medica Foundation, Washington, DC, 1977.

Brown, J., Robertson, L., Kosa, J., & Alpert, J. A study of general practice in Massachusetts. *Journal of the American Medical Association,* 216:301–306, 1971.

Cassata, D., & Kirkman-Liff, B. Mental health activities of family physicians. *Journal of Family Practice,* 12:683–692, 1981.

Coleman, J., & Patrick, D. Integrating mental health services into primary medical care. *Medical Care,* 14:654–661, 1976.

Coleman, J., & Patrick, D. Psychiatry and general health care. *American Journal of Public Health,* 68:451–457, 1978.

Cooper, B. Psychiatry and the general practitioner. *World Health Organization Chronicle,* 28:65–70, 1974.

Cooperstock, R. Some factors involved in increased prescribing of psychotropic drugs. In R. Cooperstock (Ed.), *Social Aspects of the Medical Use of Psychotropic Drugs* (pp. 21–34). Ontario: Addiction Research Foundation, 1974.

Davies, B. Psychiatric illness in general hospital clinics. *Postgraduate Medical Journal,* 40:15–18, 1964.

Eastwood, M. & Trevalyan, M. Relationships between physical and psychiatric disorder. *Psychological Medicine,* 2:363–372, 1972.

Eastwood, M. *The Relation Between Physical and Mental Illness.* Toronto: University of Toronto Press, 1975.

Eastwood, M. Screening for psychiatric disorders. *Psychological Medicine,* 1:197–205, 1971.

Enelow, A. Prevention of medical disorder: The role of the general practitioner. *California Medicine,* 104:16–21, 1966.

Engel, G. The need for a new medical model: A challenge for biomedicine. *Science,* 196:129–136, 1977.

Fink, R., Goldensohn, S., Shapiro, S., & Daily, E. Changes in family doctors' services for emotional disorders after addition of psychiatric treatment to a prepaid group practice program. *Medical Care,* 7:209–224, 1969.

Fink, R., Goldensohn, S., Shapiro, S., & Daily, E. Treatment of patients designated by family doctors as having emotional problems. *American Journal of Public Health,* 57:1550–1564, 1967.

Fink, R., Shapiro, S., & Goldensohn, S. Family physician referrals for psychiatric consultation and patient initiative in seeking care. *Social Science and Medicine,* 4:273–291, 1970.

Fink, R., & Shapiro, S. Patterns of medical care related to mental illness. *Journal of Health and Human Behavior,* 7:98–105, 1966.

France, R., Waddington, W., & Haupt, J. Referral of patients from primary care physicians to a community mental health center. *Journal of Nervous and Mental Diseases,* 166:594–598, 1978.

Gardner, A., Peterson, J., & Hall, D. A survey of general practitioners referrals to a psychiatric out-patient service. *British Journal of Psychiatry,* 124:536–541, 1974.

Glasser, M., Duggan, T., & Hoffman, W. Obstacles to utilization of prepaid mental health care. *American Journal of Psychiatry,* 137:710–715, 1975.

Goldberg, D., & Blackwell, B. Psychiatric illness in general practice. A detailed study using a new method of case identification. *British Medical Journal,* 2:434–443, 1970.

Goldberg, I., Krantz, G., & Locke, B. Effecting a short-term outpatient psychiatric therapy benefit in the utilization of medical services in a prepaid group practice medical program. *Medical Care,* 8:419–428, 1970.

Goldberg, I., Regier, D., McInenny, T., Pless, I., & Roghmann, K. The role of the pediatrician in the delivery of mental health services to children. *Pediatrics,* 63:898–909, 1979.

Group for the Advancement of Psychiatry. Committee on Public Education. *Medical Practices and Psychiatry: The Import of Changing Demands. Report No. 58.* New York: Mental Health Materials Center, 1964.

Hall, R., Gardner, E., Popkins, M., LeCann, A., & Stickney, S. Unrecognized physical illness prompting psychiatric admissions: A prospective study. *American Journal of Psychiatry,* 138:629–635, 1981.

Hankin, J., & Oktay, J. *Mental Disorder and Primary Medical Care: An Analytical Review of the Literature.* (DHEW Publication No. ADM 78-661). Washington, DC: U.S. Government Printing Office, 1979.

Harr, E., Green, H., Hyamz, L., & Jaffe, J. Varied needs of primary physicians for psychiatric resources. II. Subjective factors. *Psychosomatics,* 13:255–262, 1972.

Haupt, J., Orleans, C., George, L., & Brodie, H. The role of psychiatric and behavioral factors in the practice of medicine. *American Journal of Psychiatry,* 137:37–47, 1980.

Hopkins, P., & Cooper, B. Psychiatric referral from a general practice. *British Journal of Psychiatry,* 115:1163–1174, 1969.

Hull, J. Psychiatric referrals in general practice. *Archives of General Psychiatry,* 36:406–408, 1979.

Kaeser, A., & Cooper, B. The psychiatric patient, the general practitioner, and the outpatient clinic: An operational study and a review. *Psychological Medicine,* 1:312–305, 1971.

Katon, W., Williamson, P., & Ries, R. A prospective study of 60 consecutive psychiatric consultations in a family medicine clinic. *Journal of Family Practice,* 13:47–55, 1981.

Kaufman, M., & Bernstein, S. A psychiatric evaluation of the private patient. Study of a thousand cases from a consultation service. *Journal of the American Medical Association,* 163:108–111, 1957.

Kessel, H. The neurotic in general practice. *The Practitioner,* 194:636–641, 1965.

Lerner, R., Blackwell, B. The GP as a psychiatric community resource. *Community Mental Health Journal,* 11:3–9, 1975.

Lipowski, Z. Review of consultation psychiatry and psychosomatic medicine. II. Clinical aspects. *Psychosomatic Medicine,* 29:201–224, 1967.

Locke, B., & Gardner, E. Psychiatric disorders among patients of general practitioners and internists. *Public Health Reports,* 84:167–173, 1969.

Locke, B., Krantz, G., & Kramer, M. Psychiatric need and demand in a prepaid group practice program. *American Journal of Public Health,* 56:895–904, 1966.

Morrill, R. The future for mental health in primary health care programs. *American Journal of Psychiatry,* 135:1351–1355, 1978.

Parker, A. Dimensions of primary care: Blueprints for change. In S. Andreopoulos (Ed.), *Primary Care: Where Medicine Fails* (pp. 15–77). New York: John Wiley & Sons, 1974.

Parry, H., Balter, M., Mellinger, G., Cisin, I., & Manheimer, D. National patterns of psychotherapeutic drug use. *Archives of General Psychiatry,* 28:769–783, 1973.

Patrick, D., Eagle, J., & Coleman, J. Primary care treatment of emotional problems in an HMO. *Medical Care,* 16:47–60, 1978.

Raft, D. How to refer a reluctant patient to a psychiatrist. *American Family Physician,* 7:109–114, 1973.

Regier, D., Goldberg, I., & Taube, C. The de facto U.S. mental health services system. *Archives of General Psychiatry,* 35:685–693, 1978.

Robertson, N. Variations in referral patterns to the psychiatric services by general practitioners. *Psychological Medicine,* 9:355–364, 1979.

Roessler, R., & Greenfield, N. Incidence of somatic disease in psychiatric patients. *Psychosomatic Medicine,* 23:413–419, 1961.

Rosen, G., Kleinman, A., Katon, W. Somatization in family practice: A biopsychosocial approach. *Journal of Family Practice,* 14:493–502, 1982.

Rosen, B., Locke, B., Goldberg, I., & Babigian, H. Identification of emotional disturbances in patients seen in general medicine clinics. *Hospital and Community Psychiatry,* 23:364–470, 1972.

Shemo, J. Primary care management of mental illness: Medication as a tool. *Southern Medical Journal,* 77:1010–1019, 1984.

Shepherd, M., Cooper, B., Brown, A., & Kalton G. *Psychiatric Illness in General Practice.* London: Oxford University Press, 1966.

Shepherd, M. The general practice research unit at the Institute of Psychiatry. *Psychological Medicine,* 3:525–529, 1973.

Shortell, S., & Daniels, R. Relationships between internists and psychiatrists in fee-for-service practice: An empirical examination. *Medical Care,* 12:229–240, 1974.

Smith, H. Psychiatry in medicine: Intra- or inter-professional relationships? *American Journal of Sociology,* 63:285–289, 1957.

Solow, C. Psychotropic drugs in somatic disorders. *International Journal of Psychiatry in Medicine,* 6:267–282, 1975.

Stanford, B. Counseling: A prime area for family doctors. *American Family Physician,* 5(5):183–185, 1972.

Stoeckle, J., Zola, I., Davidson, G. The quantity and significance of psychological distress in medical patients: Some preliminary observations about the decision to seek medical aid. *Journal of Chronic Diseases,* 17:969–970, 1964.

Stoudemire A, Thompson T, Mitchell W, Grant R.: Family physicians' perceptions of psychosocial disorders. Survey report and education implications. *International Journal of Psychiatry in Medicine,* 12:281–287, 1982-1983.

Temperling, J. Psychotherapy in the setting of a general medical practice. *British Journal of Medical Psychology,* 51:139–145, 1978.

Tischler, G., Henisz, J., Myers, J., & Buswell, P. Utilization of mental health services. I. Patienthood and the prevalence of symptomatology in the community. *Archives of General Psychiatry,* 32:411–418, 1975.

U.S. Department of Health, Education, and Welfare. Public Health Service. *National Ambulatory Care Survey 1973 Summary.* (Publication No. HRA 76-1772). Hyattesville, Maryland: National Center for Health Statistics, 1975.

Wanderman, L. *Physician Distribution and Medical Licensure in the U.S., 1978.* Chicago: American Medical Association, 1979.

Weiss, T., Freeborn, D., & Lamb, S. Use of mental health services by poverty and nonpoverty members of a prepaid group practice plan. *Health Services Reports,* 88:654–662, 1973.

World Health Organization. *Psychiatry and Primary Medical Care. Report on a Working Group Convened by the Regional Office for Europe of the World Health Organization,* Oslo, April 10-13, 1973. Copenhagen: Author.

Wylon, L., & Weiner, L. Involving general practitioners in community mental health. *Hospital and Community Psychiatry,* 18:17–20, 1967.

Zung, W., MaGill, M., Moore, J., & George, D. Recognition and treatment of depression in a family medicine practice. *Journal of Clinical Psychiatry,* 44:3–6, 1983.

5

PROBLEMS FOR MENTAL HEALTH PROVIDERS

Interfaces

Recent rapid changes in social and economic values have called into question how psychiatrists, other physicians, psychologists, social workers, and psychiatric nurses can relate to each other. Thus, a new look at our boundaries is in order.

Interfaces Between Mental Health Disciplines

Appended to this Report are chapters authored by three consultants to the Committee on Governmental Agencies from the disciplines of psychology, social work, and nursing. These consultants joined with us in 1979 and participated in our deliberations. Each contributed a chapter that, by agreement, stands unedited by GAP members as the studied opinion of each professional on the definition, training requirements, strengths, and weaknesses of his or her respective professional group. Chapter 4, on the primary care sector's contributions to mental health care, is included in the body of the Report. The chapter on primary care and the appendices are of significance to the main theme of this Report, the future of psychiatry, since these sections address the opinions and identities of those professional groups that most actively interact with psychiatry in its evaluation and care of patients.

In eliciting opinions about functions of the major mental health disciplines, there is a tendency for representatives of each discipline to idealize its members. The psychiatrist is described as an exemplary primary physician, neurologist, broad-based diagnostician, psychopharmacologist, psychoanalyst, family therapist, group therapist, and behavior modification specialist. The psychologist, psychiatric social worker, and psychiatric nurse, similarly, declare that they can diagnose illness, provide all of the psychotherapies, as well as make use of the unique skills of their respective disciplines. It is implicit that all are imaginative teachers and supervisors, competent administrators, and totally at home in a hospital or clinic setting. All are free of idiosyncrasies and have the flexibility and charisma leadership on a psychiatric inpatient unit. The truth is, of course, that wide variations exist among individual mental health professionals, and the concept of attributing explicit skills to any discipline must be modified when one deals with specific individuals in a particular setting.

Each discipline has argued that its members' unique backgrounds offer something special: psychiatrists claim the capacity of ultimate medical responsibility; psychologists claim to be the "best prepared" by training; social workers, with their knowledge of family and community resources, offer "psychotherapy plus"; and nurses offer their integration of biopsychosocial knowledge and a caring tradition. One additional paradoxical feature is that all disciplines define their areas of uniqueness, but tend to disparage these special skills by emphasizing that their profession is in no way confined by its unique aspects.

While the appendices are unedited by the Committee, we feel that their integration into the theme of this Report requires some commentary.

Psychology. We are concerned about our consultants' advocacy for a *problem-oriented approach* to treatment as preferable to a diagnostic (medical) approach. Although general medicine and psychiatry have experimented with that approach for over a decade (Weed, 1968), our experience has been that, for many psychiatric patients, such an approach tends to discourage an integration of problems into patterns or syndromes that provide the comprehensive viewpoint needed to arrive at treatment plans that best effect change. For example, a patient may have a "problem" of low self-esteem because of recurrent depressions, an anxiety disorder, the relationship-forming difficulty inherent in schizophrenia, or developmental or characterologic problems with trust, intimacy, etc. The treatment of each of these causes of low self-esteem is quite different. We believe that often the problem-oriented approach results in oversimplification of the many-layered conditions against which our patients struggle.

The Committee is disturbed by our consultants' implication that the only real impediments to psychology's function as a fully autonomous and comprehensive profession in the treatment of mental illness lies in external restraints on psychologists' ability to function essentially like psychiatrists. We maintain that such restrictions have a legitimate basis in the realities of the training of the respective groups.

Two examples that our psychologist consultant mentions in this regard are the prescription of psychotropic drugs and the granting of hospital privileges. In regard to *psychotropic drugs*, we maintain that the appropriate use of somatic interventions in mental illness is a complex process and requires medical training in its totality. The pervasive and intricate interactions among bodily systems require knowledge of the whole of medicine to competently prescribe and monitor psychiatric medications, just as to prescribe cardiac medications. Because of the increasing array and complexity of psychopharmacologic therapy, the amount of time spent in rigorous training and supervised experience in handling these powerful agents has increased dramatically in almost all psychiatric residency programs. The simple addition of a few "courses" in psychopharmacology to the training of a psychologist would not, in our opinion, allow competency in this area.

We see a similar paradox in the area of *hospital privileges*. The issue of hospitalization is complex and has been further complicated by recent economic pressures to severely limit hospital use. The privilege of hospital admission carries with it great responsibilities for the well-being of patients. Hospitalization today is typically indicated only when the patient is very ill, when diagnostic issues are highly complex, or when the proposed treatment carries the potential for side effects that must be monitored closely. The psychiatrist is clearly the best-equipped professional to manage a comprehensive examination and treatment of patients under those circumstances. We do not believe that the addition of a primary care physician's physical exam to the evaluation of a psychologist is equivalent to the assessment and care given by a psychiatrist.

There are, however, psychiatrists who have limited their practice to office or outpatient techniques and who are thereby no longer up-to-date on hospital treatment modalities. Often they refer their patients needing inpatient care to hospital-oriented psychiatrists, and we endorse this approach. This issue of "primary psychiatric expertise" will be addressed further in Chapter 7.

Our consultant's argument that psychologists should have full hospital privileges because they serve on the faculties of medical schools is faulty. Many individuals from various professions are on medical school faculties without expecting to function in the role of physician. Examples include sociologists, cardiac physiologists, radiation physicists, and orthopedic appliance specialists.

Our consultant of psychology notes the lack of the experience of responsibility for life and death decision making as a relative weakness for psychologists, which could be alleviated if psychologists were put in such positions while in training. We doubt that the training of psychologists could be so easily rectified. Critical and ultimate responsibility is a function that the psychiatrist has painfully developed throughout eight years of medical training and residency and is integral to that experience; it cannot be easily grafted onto other orientations of training.

While we agree with our consultant that psychology has an identity as both a science and a profession, we question his contention that this is unique. All branches of the medical profession have their roots in a rigorous scientific tradition. This is evidenced by the years of training in the sciences required for a medical background and by the tradition of basic and clinical research conducted at medical schools, hospitals, and other medical setting. The recent, almost unmanageable explosion of scientific articles documenting psychiatric research is as exciting as it is impressive (see Chapter 6).

At a time when psychiatric training is becoming ever more medically rigorous, and the knowledge psychiatrists are expected to master is exponentially increasing, it is paradoxical that groups without a comparable background in training and experience would claim the ability to function equivalently. In our opinion, psychologists would service the public interest by being very clear in their public self-identity that they are not psychiatrically/medically trained and by accepting responsibility for obtaining psychiatric input when they are caring for a patient who may have a mental illness. While they may choose not to function within a medical model, since their training is not relevant to this model, they should recognize the value and necessity of this approach for mentally ill patients. Thus while we agree that many psychologists are well trained to practice psychotherapy, we hold that the diagnosis of illness and the prescription of appropriate treatment goes far beyond the practice of psychotherapy. The reciprocal responsibility of the psychiatrist is to respect the expertise of the psychologist and not displace him or her as primary therapist when ongoing psychiatric expertise is unnecessary.

Social work. Many of the concerns the Committee would express regarding this chapter, if taken in isolation, would be a repetition of issues noted above. Several areas specific to this chapter, however, may stand consideration. First, we feel that the claim to a *biopsychosocial orientation* in social work is weak. Certainly the attractiveness of this perspective, as outlined by numerous authors (Engel, 1980), is so strong as to make the use of the term almost mandatory. Nonetheless, the two years of postgraduate training required for attaining an M.S.W., while sufficient to introduce the importance of biological factors in the function of individuals, is clearly not adequate to allow any but rudimentary skills in evaluating and integrating these factors. To make an analogy, knowing that engineering skills are essential for building a bridge is not equivalent to personally having those skills. While some social workers obtain doctoral degrees in social work, little of the additional training involves the basic biological sciences.

We find the contention that social work provides "psychotherapy plus," because of the integration of family and social systems data, questionable in that good psychotherapeutic understanding and technique has always demanded a knowledge of the matrix in which the individual functions. In medical practice one includes the family and social structure when treating a juvenile diabetic or an asthmatic patient, just as one does when treating a young schizophrenic or bulimic patient or a suicidal adolescent.

Psychiatric mental health nursing. Unfortunately, the chapter (Appendix C) does not clearly distinguish between nurses with master's-or doctoral-level degrees and the larger group of nurses with B.S. or lesser degrees. Since the most frequent contact between a psychiatric nurse and a psychiatrist, or other mental health professional, involves a nurse with less than a master's training, it would have been useful to have had this group specifically addressed.

Our consultant states that psychiatric/mental health nursing is *based on theory and models* rather than on procedures. The author seems to criticize other areas of nursing for tending to be more pragmatic or "guided by principles rather than theories." One could understand that, if a field seeks true autonomy, a lack of theoretical base might be perceived as a weakness and development of theories as a goal. Furthermore, labeling that goal as an inherent "strength" may encourage colleagues to seek a stronger theoretical base. If one accepts our premise that the needs of psychiatric patients are best met by a differentiation of roles among the groups that provide care, then it would seem that the nursing tradition of hands-on, practical, pragmatic involvement would be central to their contribution. To move away from this model would leave a serious gap in the services needed by the mentally ill.

The GAP Committee finds itself in disagreement with our consultant's description of the unique characteristics of nursing. First, we disagree that the "core mental health professionals share roughly the *same body of knowledge.*" The lengthy training obtained by a psychiatrist should lead to a considerable incremental advance in knowledge. As it stands, our consultants statement would be analogous to saying that an operating room nurse shares the same body of knowledge as a neurosurgeon. Both work in the same area and do vital and independently important work, but their knowledge, training, and experience are hardly the same. Our consultant overstates the case by saying that nurses "are able to determine whether or not a given behavioral disturbance might have organic underpinnings." While nurses are more familiar with organic disturbances than social workers, and often more so than psychologists, they are hardly "able to determine" this issue. We likewise disagree that the "use of biological as well as psychological therapies in providing holistic health care" is unique to nursing. While this hopefully is a characteristic of psychiatric nursing, surely it is true of psychiatry but at quite a different level of proficiency.

Our consultant states that nurses need not be admonished to *"first do no harm,"* as do physicians. We feel she is underestimating the influence of nursing interaction and decisions on the well-being of patients. The actions of nurses, the care they provide, and the attitude with which it is done, the verbal and nonverbal messages that they give patients and families, their support or obstruction of the physician's treatment plan, all have a powerful impact on the patient. Since an intervention powerful enough to have a positive effect inexorably carries the potential for harm, we would caution that nurses too need to heed this time-tested dictum, as indeed most do.

The author of the appendix on psychiatric nursing is not as adamant as the psychologist about the issue of autonomy in practice, but there is the statement that nurses "insist on the right to determine the dimensions of their practice in an autonomous fashion." To the extent that this implies the ability to diagnose illness and prescribe treatment by the growing number of nurses in independent private practice, we voice the same disagreement and concerns previously stated.

The Health–Mental Health Interface

Chapter 4 describes the interface between primary care physicians and mental health professionals. We noted that most patients seen in the primary care sector with a diagnosis of a mental illness tend to remain in that sector and that some of them do not receive optimum care. Of those who are offered a referral to a psychiatrist, many refuse to accept the referral or simply do not appear at the psychiatrist's office. Factors that hinder the referral process include psychiatry's limited acceptance as a medical specialty, the patient's fear of mental illness, the primary physician's fear of "insulting " his patient by suggesting a psychiatric referral, and the referring physician's frustration at being unable to find an organic basis for the patient's symptoms. These factors frequently lead to the referral being experienced by the patients as either a personal rejection or as proof that their complaints were not legitimate.

Most difficult to manage are patients who tend to deny their illness or who resist the psychiatric implications of their disorders. These include patients with character disorders, drug and alcohol abuse problems, and some somatization disorders such as chronic pain syndromes. Attempts at referral that the patient experiences as rejection will serve only to increase the number, severity, and intensity of the patients' symptoms and demands (Bowlby, 1973; Kolb, 1982).

A collaborative relationship with a psychiatrist can be helpful to the primary-care physician in developing strategies for management of patients within the primary-care setting. Patient preparation for referral is also a critical determinant of its success. Psychiatric referral is often more acceptable to patients when the referring physician views the psychiatrist as a medical colleague with specialty expertise (Roft, 1973; Smith, 1957). The psychiatrist must also reinforce this impression by his demeanor with the patient (McCue, 1982; Schubert, 1978). The willingness of the primary-care physician to maintain a relationship with the patient following referral is helpful in obviating the patient's apprehension of being excluded from the medical care system.

Both patients and physicians conceptualize a significant amount of the mental health treatment given in primary-care settings as the management of stress or stress-related complications. While such a formulation has the benefit of being less threatening to patients and their families, it has the major drawback of being so broad and scientifically ill defined as to offer little guidance regarding either prognosis or treatment. Psychotropic medications are useful in stress management to the extent that the patient's physiologic or emotional response to stress has been in the form of a recognizable mental illness. Thus, accurate diagnosis is the cornerstone of such intervention (Imboden & Urbaitis, 1978; Shemo, 1984).

Liaison psychiatrists consulting with primary care physicians often have difficulty getting reimbursed for their time because insurance companies tend to pay for direct patient care only. Furthermore, there is no precedent within the medical community for consulting with a psychiatrist about what is perceived as one's personal difficulties with patients. Nevertheless, psychiatrists have been useful and cost-effective in helping provide better primary care for medical/surgical patients with concurrent mental illness (see p. 104–109).

There is also an economic side. Because of conceptual problems as well as difficulty in obtaining funding for the treatment of mental illness from the Congress, the federal government has traditionally separated funding for mental health care from general health care. Where integration of mental health knowledge into that of general medicine is essential, such as in remote areas where all health resources are scarce or where patients in any setting present with combined health-mental health symptoms, this separation has created unnecessary problems. However, attempts at the integration of general health care and mental health care are increasing. Among other factors, this trend recognizes that general health care settings deal with large numbers of deinstitutionalized mentally ill patients living in communities. Coleman and Patrick (1976) conclude that for an integrated plan to succeed, it should ideally start with the opening of the new health center, thereby escaping the inertia that has caused so many programs in more established settings to fail. Solid administrative support and a collaborative effort by both primary care physicians and psychiatric staff are essential to increase the effectiveness of mental health services (Cooper Harwin, Delpa, & Shepherd, 1975). Where this

has occurred, primary care physicians have identified larger numbers of patients with emotional problems, have kept more of them
within the primary provider's active caseload, and prescribed
psychotropic drugs more appropriately, reflecting a higher quality
of care (Fink, Goldensohn, Shapiro, & Daily, 1969).

Funding for the treatment of mental illness is difficult. Unfortunately, patients who have experienced mental illness are politically weak and, in addition, do not readily attract nonprofit health
agency sponsorship, such as the American Heart Association. In
the 1950s when coalitions of mental health advocates and providers, along with their state and national organizations, demanded
adequate funding for the mentally ill, they met with moderate
success. This coalition was seriously weakened during the recent
era when some of our own colleagues considered mental illness a
myth and when many mental health associations were concentrat-
ing their efforts on "patient rights" issues rather than lobbying for
more support for treatment. While we see a potential benefit for
the government to combine general health (illness) clinics with
mental health (illness) clinics, as is now done in many private
settings and hospitals, there remains the risk that, ultimately, depression and schizophrenia cannot compete successfully in the marketplace with heart attacks, stroke, and cancer.

The Mental Health–Mental Illness Paradox

Leighton points out the paradox that the term "mental health,"
substituted early in this century for "mental illness," also serves to
deny its existence. Furthermore, the organic underpinnings of
mental illness were, and still are, deemphasized by advocates of
"mental health" (1982, pp. 28, 74). As a more recent example of this
paradox, for over three decades the community "mental health"
movement strove to deliver "primary prevention" of mental illness,
in an attempt to duplicate in this field what had been so successful
in the public health field earlier this century in preventing infectious disease. When the results of relatively generous funding for
primary prevention in community mental health centers (CMHCs)
was reviewed in the late 1970s, results were disappointing. NIMH

and local funders directed CMHCs to focus on direct treatment of patients with mental illness in order to maintain public credibility and support. The "mental health" providers were too often focused on better education, better parenting, and restructuring the community and its social organization. Actual treatment of the mentally ill was relabled "tertiary prevention" in a curious contortion of words that also tended to underplay the reality of mental illness. It is no wonder, then, that mentally ill people are overlooked. The denial of "illness" and of biological parameters was a factor that inhibited a broader perspective, including a search for the knowledge of the causes or precursors of major mental illness that could be addressed either through prevention or treatment.

On the other hand, the term "mental illness" still conveys such a confusingly broad range of conditions that communication, research, planning, goal setting, and funding are impaired. "Mental illness" still tends to conjure wildly emotional reactions from the public ("stigma"), and until recently has lacked the scientific basis that inspires trust and funding for either research or treatment (Leighton, 1982, pp. 6–16).

From the viewpoint of third-party funders, mental health professionals have not been effective in separating treatment of mental illness from helping unhappy clients cope with "normal" problems in living or from creating a growth experience for otherwise healthy and functioning individuals. All mental health professionals are clearly involved across this spectrum and would like health (illness) insurance to pay for all their services. To further complicate matters, many schools and colleges, nonprofit activity-oriented organizations (such as the YMCA), and health groups also address the healthier end of the spectrum with educational programs. Perhaps health and mental health education should be taught (and funded) by schools rather than by clinics.

Autonomy Under Siege

Professional autonomy is clearly a major issue for all disciplines. The psychiatric discipline, without concurrence from the others, believes that it should function as the preferred diagnostician for all cases requesting treatment by *any* mental health professional in which there is a suspicion of mental illness. Psychiatrists argue that the recent knowledge of effective pharmacological interventions for many depressed or anxiety-ridden patients and the ever-present specter of patients receiving ineffective psychotherapy for an undiagnosed but treatable medical ailment support the case that only they, with their broad medical background, can address these diagnostic decisions adequately. They feel that the length of psychiatric training (including medical school), as well as the medical tradition, further supports the notion that they should be not only diagnosticians, but also supervisors of other mental health professionals in those cases where a psychiatric viewpoint regarding mental illness is an important factor.

Other disciplines challenge these claims of special competence. Psychologists, with claims of long-recognized skills in diagnostic testing, study of scientific psychology, and tradition of self-policing, see little merit in arguments for psychiatric dominance. They claim that they may have more years of psychological didactic training and work experience during their training period than some psychiatrists. Social workers, experienced in sorting out social, economic, familial, interpersonal, and intrapersonal problems for their clients since the early 1930s, make a case for both primacy and autonomy. Master's-level psychiatric nurses claim both a long nursing tradition of responsibility for the most seriously ill and of continuity of care for institutionalized patients. They also maintain that their biopsychosocial systems background obviates the need for the expertise of a psychiatrist, except when requested.

Autonomy Versus Supervision

There is little controversy that supervision is an essential part of training of all mental health professionals. But there is less consensus that supervision should be required after the training period is completed. State licensing boards (page 25) take the stance that if you have graduated from the appropriate schools and can pass the licensing examination, you are prepared to serve the public safely without additional supervision. Our psychologist consultant decries any *forced* supervision of one discipline by another and claims that, particularly in clinical evaluation and psychotherapy, the psychologist is the expert anyway. Our nurse consultant points out that psychiatric nurses traditionally received supervision in psychotherapy from other disciplines, but that this tradition was a factor in the profession's low self-esteem. Thus the new master's-level mental health nurses hope to assume the supervisory role.

Those of us who supervise, or have been supervised, know that the most vexing supervisory problems occur when the person supervised is unaware that there is a problem. Artemus Ward (1834–1867) is supposed to have said, "It ain't the things we don't know that hurt us. It's the things we do know that ain't so!" Can mental health professionals be taught to know when they need to seek help? Can one measure competence to supervise? Should the supervisory hierarchy be based on clinical experience? years of training? on specific training? on medical training? Descriptions of all four mental health disciplines stress the importance of academic degrees and years of training within their respective disciplines. Is there, therefore, a responsibility of more highly trained disciplines toward those who are less well trained? Perhaps supervision across disciplines should be limited to specific techniques. The issues of peer supervision and even peer review (often of written records only) raise similar questions.

While organized settings generally impose a supervisory hierarchy, private practice by its very nature is not supervised. Some private mental health professionals do seek out colleagues with whom to share their therapeutic problems and should be encouraged to do so. However, the majority probably do not. Two of the advantages of the private practice model are autonomy of the practitioner and privacy for the patient. How can these be preserved under a system of forced supervision or peer review? We need more documented experience in these important areas.

Autonomy Versus Controlled Access to Treatment

The question of who controls access to mental health professionals is now posed not only in organized settings, but also in the private sector. As noted in Chapter 2, the California state legislation recently wrote laws to permit private health insurance carriers, such as Blue Cross, to contract with specific provider organizations for health care using specified predetermined fees. Some of the resulting preferred provider organizations (PPOs) have designated primary care physicians as the only persons who may refer a patient to specialists, including psychiatrists and other mental health professionals. Most "mentally ill adults" (MIAs) funded under California's Medicaid (Medi-Cal) must also go through the primary care gate. Medicare is toying with the same notions.

On page 24 we suggest that the tradition of independent private practice has the potential for unwise use of society's resources because of the lack of a triage system to look after the needs of those who cannot afford private care, who cannot choose wisely, or who choose not to use any system. Chapter 2 documents growing numbers of these ill nonpatients. Organized settings generally sort out which patients should go to which practitioner for what service, but there is no similar system in private practice. There is some evidence that "gatekeepers" are expensive and that patients who can perform their own triage should go directly to a dermatologist or a psychiatrist or social worker, without the added delay and expense of seeing a general practitioner (Moore, Martin & Richardson, 1983). We have noted the limited sophistication of some primary care practitioners about mental illness (pages 66–71) and will describe the "offset effect" (pages 104–109) that points out the lower overall costs when mental health care is integrated with traditional medical care (in some organized settings). But issues of remaining stigma associated with mental illness, on the one hand, and the desire for autonomy by health professionals, on the other, make such integration difficult.

In Chapter 3 we recommend that psychiatrists be involved in initial diagnosis, treatment plans, and ongoing responsibility for patients with a mental illness. How would one mandate such a "gatekeeping" system, particularly in private practice? The insurance industry, CHAMPUS, Medicaid, and some state legislatures (under "freedom of choice" legislation) are encouraging the growth and direct payment of numerous old and new mental health professionals and counselors on the theory that competition will eventually drive down costs. On the other hand, there is some evidence that more providers mean more total costs, based on the fiscally frightening prospect that the market demand for mental health services is relatively unlimited. Again, we are short of knowledgeable answers.

Autonomy Versus the Marketplace

During the early days of the community mental health movement, Congress was relatively generous with funding; there was more mental health work than could be performed, and the various mental health disciplines were rapidly growing and working together to meet the expanding work load. In the private sector the entire health care industry grew by leaps and bounds, safely funded by private and governmental medical insurance that paid essentially whatever providers said was the cost. Times have obviously changed. The recurrence of territorial battles between disciplines may mean that the field is now saturated or that funds are drying up—probably both.

Mental health is big business today (Bittker, 1985). The growth of health maintenance organizations (HMOs) and preferred provider organizations (PPOs) and the entry of large, for profit hospital corporations into the arena of psychiatric treatment, herald a major change in the manner in which psychiatrists will practice medicine in the next decades. Yet psychiatrists are just now becoming interested in marketing their services. With a clear limit to the amount of money our society is willing to spend on any health care, psychiatrists will most likely not decide who gets paid for what services. Decisions regarding which clinicians will be hired, whom they will treat for which conditions, and how much they will be reimbursed for their services are being made today by politicians and businessmen, not clinicians. If the marketplace decides our future, as is the case in competitive industries, mental health treatment may be performed by the cheapest, least-trained persons available, or the size of one's pocketbook may determine the quality of treatment one can obtain. Representatives from industry, government bureaucrats, insurance actuaries, and mental health professionals are discussing these issues singly and in groups, but the answers still escape us.

Automomy Versus External Regulations

Psychologists oppose regulation by the medical establishment and complain about exclusion from hospital staffs by the Joint Commission for the Accreditation of Hospitals, (JCAH). Psychiatrists have been vocal in opposing the intrusion into their practices by insurance companies and by the government and its judicial representatives. Yet absolute autonomy is a fantasy and is not necessarily a good thing, particularly where quality is an issue. We have seen examples of successful regulation, such as imposition of controls over medical schools after the Flexner report in 1914. The question, then, is one of balance. Who should decide competence to practice alone? How should claims to autonomy in practice be assessed? How costly will regulations be to administer? Historically, antitrust legislation and governmental regulations have developed when an industry became too big, noncompetitive, and a threat to the general welfare. That is happening now in the health field, and the consequences will affect both patients and practitioners.

Special Problems with Psychotherapy

The Committee, through the process of deliberation with our consultants, was struck on several occasions by the differences in our conceptualizations about psychotherapy. Historically, physicians with special interest in mental illnesses were very much in the "mainstream" of the empirical, deductive and scientific tradition of medical progress. By the early part of the twentieth century, however, clinical advancement was stymied by the limitations of the available methodology, and psychiatry turned toward a more inductive and theoretical model, from which derived much of dynamic theory and psychotherapeutic technique. As Freud pointed out, however, this approach was designed to allow the development of treatment strategies as an interim measure until further advances in knowledge could foster a revival in our process of establishing basic, verifiable understanding of etiologic factors (Meissner, 1980). The gains made during this period were major and must not be forgotten or discarded. Nonetheless, there has been an exponential growth in our knowledge base, and this new data must, and is, being integrated into our repertoire of treatment stategies.

During the years of the "theoretical era" in psychiatry, a model of psychotherapy developed which was incorporated, and in some cases elaborated and refined, by groups outside of the medical tradition. This model has subsequently been applied to a wide variety of human situations, both by psychiatrists and other groups involved in mental health treatment, with varying degrees of success. Thus, during this era, there was a degree of convergence in therapeutic methodologies and therefore in the identities of psychiatry and the other groups. Increasingly, however, differences are becoming more apparent. As the array of differentially efficacious modalities of treatment expands, the necessity for comprehensive diagnosis, rather than, or in addition to, dynamic formulation, becomes clear.

There are also problems with the term "psychotherapy" itself. In Chapter 6 we show evidence that specific therapists from various mental health disciplines can provide effective psychotherapy for selected problems. Yet the term "psychotherapy" has become so diluted during the rapid growth of mental health providers that it has lost credibility with most funders, in spite of our observation that skillful psychotherapy can be lifesaving for some patients with a severe mental illness. How long can third-party reimbursement for generic psychotherapy continue, if a growing number of practitioners, no matter how well trained, are demanding their fair share, without breaking the funding institutions that are primarily identified with health (read "illness") care?

The major costs of today's health care stem from lengthy or intensive hospital care, not psychiatric office visits. Yet the specter of unlimited, "unnecessary" psychotherapy appears to haunt the insurance policymakers out of proportion to the fiscal impact (see pp. 104–107). Continued loss of third-party reimbursements would compromise nearly all current mental health treatment. *We recommend that psychotherapy for mental illness be considered an essential part of its treatment and that it should be reimbursed to the same extent as treatment of any other illness.*

References

Bittker, T.E. The industrialization of American psychiatry, *American Journal of Psychiatry* 142:2, 1985.

Bowlby, J. *Attachment and Loss*. New York: Basic Books, 1973.

Coleman, J., & Patrick, D. Integrating mental health services into primary medical care. *Medical Care*, 14:654–661, 1976.

Cooper, B., Harwin, B., Delpa, C., & Shepherd, M. Mental health care in the community: An evaluative study. *Psychological Medicine*, 5:372–380, 1975.

Engel, G. The clinical application of the biopsychosocial model. *American Journal of Psychiatry*, 137:535–544, 1980.

Fink, R., Goldensohn, S., Shapiro, S., & Daily, E.F. Changes in family doctors' services for emotional disorders after addition of psychiatric treatment to a prepaid group practice program. *Medical Care*, 7(3):209–224, 1969.

Imboden, J., & Urbaitis, J. *Practical Psychiatry in Medicine* (pp. 248–265). New York: Appleton-Century-Crofts, 1978.

Kolb, L. Attachment behavior and pain complaints. *Psychosomatics*, 23:413–425, 1982.

Leighton, A.H. *Caring for Mentally Ill People*. New York: Cambridge University Press, 1982.

McCue, J. Psychiatric consultation to internal medicine: an internist's thoughts. *Psychosomatics*, 23:832–839, 1982.

Meissner, W. Theories of personality and psychopathology: classical psychoanalysis. In H. Kaplan, A. Freedman, & B. Saddock (Eds.), *Comprehensive Textbook of Psychiatry/III* (pp. 631–728). Baltimore: Williams & Wilkins, 1980.

Moore, S.H., Martin, D.M., & Richardson, W.C. Does the primary-care gatekeeper control the costs of health care? *New England Journal of Medicine*, 309(22):1400–1404, 1983.

Roft, D. How to refer a reluctant patient to a psychiatrist. *American Family Physician*, 7:109–114, 1973.

Schubert, D. Obstacles to effective psychiatric liaison. *Psychosomatics*, 19:283–285, 1978.

Shemo, J. Primary care management of mental illness: Medication as a tool. *Southern Medical Journal*, 77:1010–1014, 1984.

Smith, H. Psychiatry in medicine: Intra- or inter-professional relationships? *American Journal of Sociology*, 63:285–289, 1957.

Weed, L.L. Medical records that guide and teach. *New England Journal of Medicine*, 278(11):593–600, 652–657, 1968.

Section III

CHANGING TIMES

6

NEW KNOWLEDGE FOR PSYCHIATRY

The previous chapter focused on a number of problems facing psychiatrists and other professionals involved in the mental health/illness field. This chapter, in contrast, presents an overview of new knowledge gleaned from basic and clinical research, from controlled studies on the effectiveness of our treatments, and from recent reports on the epidemiology of mental illness. We particularly wish to convey a growing excitement among psychiatrists about this recent information. We suggest that the information presented brings psychiatry closer to the rest of the medical profession, without threatening the diversity of the field, and offers the hope of a more scientific approach to integrating the field.

Recent Basic and Clinical Research Findings

Psychiatry as a clinical discipline has undergone considerable change in the past 10 years. The impetus for this change has been derived from both the biological and psychodynamic ends of the biopsychosocial spectrum in which we function, and the implications, particularly for the need to integrate the field, have a major impact on all spheres.

Recent research is just beginning to affect clinical psychiatry in areas that were only of interest to researchers a few years ago. These include 1) the discovery of the endorphin and benzodiazepine receptors in the brain; 2) the advances in our understanding of the genetics of psychiatric illness in terms of the spectrum concept of illnesses, such as depression, sociopathy, and alcoholism, brought about by pedigree studies; 3) the increased awareness of the relationship between EEG abnormalities, especially in the temporal lobe areas, and psychiatric illness; 4) the increased understanding of the wide range of clinical presentations of anxiety disorders, as occurs in agoraphobia and panic disorders; and 5) the awareness that character pathology may at times be the result of other, more specific disorders, either organic or affective, occurring at critical stages of development.

Many of the most promising research findings have not yet affected routine psychiatric practices. These include 1) the PET scan correlates of schizophrenia and dementing illness; 2) the computer-assisted evaluation of CT findings in chronic psychotic states, especially schizophrenia; 3) the HLA-typing correlates of depression; and 4) the neurotransmitter correlates of violent and suicidal behavior.

Further, there have been some impressive advances in the range and uses of psychotropic drugs. These include 1) the wider use of lithium to treat a variety of affective conditions; 2) the use of carbamazapine to treat both the psychiatric complications of epileptic disorders and some treatment-resistant forms of affective and psychotic illnesses; 3) the introduction of new antidepressants with at least some potential advantages with regard to side effects; 4) the use of MAO inhibitors for atypical depressions; 5) the use of tricyclic antidepressants in chronic pain conditions; and 6) the use of tricyclic antidepressants and MAO inhibitors in the treatment of panic and agoraphobic disorders.

A third arena of new developments involves those areas of interface between psychiatry, neurology, and internal medicine. This includes greater appreciation for 1) the interaction of nociceptive and affective pathways in chronic pain conditions; 2) the psychiatric complications of the diseases of aging, especially dementing disorders; 3) the CNS complications of many of the new drugs used to treat various physical disorders, such as levodopa, cimetidine, and cancer chemotherapeutic agents; and 4) the problems inherent in the increased lifespan of patients with numerous previously fatal conditions such as lupus, Parkinson's disease, and chronic renal failure.

Advances in the psychodynamic realm are no less impressive. A thoroughgoing reevaluation of schemes of normal development in human beings, from earliest infancy until senescence, is under way. Much more observational and empirical data are now available than in the past. Efforts are under way to give more careful accounts of how constitutional endowment and psychosocial surroundings interact in development. For example, the effects of both physical and psychic trauma on maturation and symptom production are under systematic study. Promising work seeks to meld psychoanalytically inspired infant and mother observation with sophisticated neurophysiological measurements in the hope that primary prevention strategies will follow.

Theories regarding both male and female psychosexual development are undergoing continued refinement. The impact of traumata in the family, including disruptions like death, chronic illness and disability, divorce, violence, and incest are under study. There are also recent long-term and twin studies regarding what determines vulnerability for alcohol and drug abuse, what preventative measures may be taken, and what treatment may be directed both toward patients with these disorders and toward their children and grandchildren. Studies of "expressed emotion" in the families of schizophrenics and its relation to relapse may be pointing toward a powerful psychosocial influence with major impact not only on the patient's clinical state, but also on patient care costs.

These advances have demanded a greater emphasis in psychiatric training on those areas that will allow the young psychiatrist to understand and integrate the attendant theoretical and practical implications. Since it is axiomatic that any intervention that has powerful effects will also have powerful side effects, the development of the expertise need to ethically use the increasing repertoire of somatic therapies has required some degree of remedicalization in psychiatry.

Likewise, studies in anxiety disorders, phobic disorders, mood disorders, eating disorders, alcoholism, antisocial personality, and borderline personality suggest important genetic-organic factors that at times must be integrated in the overall formulations of treatment

needs along with emotional and social factors. This in no way de-
values the importance of the dynamic issues, but rather suggests that
they be conceptualized within a broader, more integrative perspective.

With many conditions what we have are not curative but amelio-
rative potentials based on emerging understanding of the natural
history of certain illnesses, in particular, human ecologies. Research
results generally do not dictate simple clinical treatment strategies,
but rather make the understanding and management of psychiatric patients more complex. Thus the psychiatrist must synthesize
more information to implement and carry out a modern treatment
plan. Psychiatry is a field of ferment as it approaches the enormously
complex human experience.

New Knowledge in Perspective

In spite of the many new findings noted above, we must conclude that the complexities of the mind and its biosocial interactions are so vast that we have just touched the surface in terms of
relatively hard, scientifically validated knowledge. Yet we as clinicians use an enormous body of "softer" knowledge and theory
learned in the classroom, in supervision, in discussions with peers,
in studying the literature, and in treating patients, which sustains us
and guides us in daily practice. Recent advances in knowledge
about mental disorders suggest an increase in the importance of
biological factors in their course and treatment. However, we must
integrate this perspective with the valuable insights from psychoanalysis, ego psychology, social psychology, learning theory, family systems, and many other fields that have permitted us to help
relieve the suffering of many patients over the past 50 years. We
often deal with the subjective and must remember that some ideas
cannot be studied or proved in the scientific laboratory but may
nonetheless be valid in practice; conversely, we cannot naively
assume that they are valid because we wish them to be. Technologi-
cal advances are opening new avenues to study the mind and brain,
but we must await the slow, painful, scientific process that will
eventually validate what is useful and what is not.

Clinical Implications

The new knowledge about depressions and about certain panic states has created an awareness that psychiatric opinion at the onset of treatment is important so that patients who might respond rapidly with the addition of medications do not spend fruitless time in psychotherapy with nonmedically oriented providers. The fact that this new knowledge is available primarily to psychiatrists changes the relationships among mental health providers. Alternatively, the prescription of an antidepressant by a primary care physician without a careful psychiatric assessment or without engaging the psychosocial aspects of the illness may be just as fruitless. Thus psychiatrists have a special responsibility to define and disseminate advances in diagnosis and treatment of the mentally ill and to employ the integrative functions unavailable to other practitioners.

A second issue concerns which practitioners should know what knowledge about mental illness. Should we train generalists or subspecialists in mental health? Who should know what is known? Behind the experiments with role blurring in CMHCs in the 1960s and 1970s was the implication that there is a body of knowledge and set of attitudes toward patients that any competent mental health professional could know and should know. An example is knowing when to be sympathetic toward some patients or firm with others. Individual talents for empathy and charisma also played prominent roles and were seen across the spectrum of professionals and nonprofessionals alike. With the proliferation of new, specialized knowledge in the field, it is expedient to encourage role differentiation among and even within disciplines so that patients can have access to informed clinical interventions.

Effectiveness and Cost-Effectiveness of Psychiatric Interventions

Clinical Effectiveness

Today the effectiveness of specific interventions for specific mental disorders should give rise to optimism. The literature documents the effectiveness of appropriately selected psychotropic agents in the treatment of the major psychotic illnesses and major depressions (Davis, 1976; Davis, Shaffer, Killian, Kinard, & Chan, 1980; Klein & Davis, 1969; Klein, Gittelman, Quitkin, & Rifkin, 1980). The clinical effectiveness of psychotherapies of varied specificity is also encouraging (Bergin, 1971; Eysenck, 1966; Rachman, 1977). *We wish to emphasize that the psychiatrist often uses medications together with some form of psychotherapy to treat patients with the major mental disorders, even though this Report presents the evidence in separate sections.*

Specific psychopharmacological therapies. The evidence supporting the clinical efficacy of the antipsychotic drugs, such as phenothiazines, butyrophenones, and thioxanthenes, in the treatment of schizophrenia is overwhelming. Klein and Davis (1969) reviewed the extensive evidence in documenting the superiority of antipsychotic drugs over placebo and sedative agents in the management of acute or recurrent schizophrenia. In 1979 Davis and associates (1980) reviewed 24 studies on maintenance therapy of schizophrenia and demonstrated the clear superiority of antipsychotics to placebo in treatments lasting at least one month. In addition, the clinical efficacy of antipsychotics in the treatment of chronic schizophrenia is no longer in question. One must keep in mind that antipsychotics relieve some of the symptoms of schizophrenia, especially the positive symptoms, and are highly useful. They rarely cure schizophrenia, however, and are best used as part of a comprehensive treatment plan including both psychological and social elements.

Tricyclic antidepressants (TCAs) have a similar role in the treatment of major depressions. Klein and Davis (1969) reviewed 65 studies comparing TCAs with placebo; 50 of these studies clearly showed the TCAs to be superior. The currently relevant questions for investigation include the following: 1) For which subgroups are the TCAs most effective? and 2) which patients may be better treated with MAO-inhibitors, lithium, ECT, or various psychotherapies?

The efficacy of lithium carbonate has been studied as an agent for the primary treatment of manic and depressive episodes of affective disorders and as a prophylactic agent for use in patients with either bipolar disorder or recurrent unipolar depression. The research literature on the use of lithium was meticulously reviewed by Klein and associates (1980). After examining seven carefully executed, double-blind, placebo-controlled studies of lithium's effect on the treatment of depression, these researchers concluded that "lithium has a therapeutic effect on depression" (p. 334). Research studies reporting on the treatment of mania were "uniformly enthusiastic about the clinical efficacy of lithium" (p. 226).

Regarding the *prophylactic* use of lithium in the management of manic-depressive illness. Davis (1976) reviewed eight studies that compared placebo with lithium using a random assignment and blind evaluation method. He concluded,

> The empirical data clearly show that lithium has quite a substantial prophylactic effect, one that is highly significant statistically and one that is consistently demonstrated in all studies. These conclusions are reinforced by the fact that several studies were collaborative and multiinstitutional and consistently demonstrated the lithium effect in the different institutions. (p. 3)

Finally, Davis (1976) and Klein and associates (1980) reviewed lithium's efficacy in the prophylaxis of recurrent depression. They concur that, in contrast to its treatment effect, lithium has a statistically significant effect in preventing relapse in recurrent unipolar depression. While Davis found that lithium has significant prophylactic effects against depression in both the bipolar and unipolar groups, Klein and associates found the evidence to be inconclusive for the prevention of recurrence of depression on patients with bipolar disorders but with the trend suggesting a "strong possibility" (p. 344) for such an effect.

General psychotherapies. Most recent studies of outcome have reported that psychotherapy is helpful. Outcome measures, however, have been difficult to assess (Epstein & Vlok,1981; Luborsky,

Singer, & Luborsky, 1975; Meltzoff & Kornreich, 1970; Smith, Glass, & Miller, 1980). In view of the difficulties involved in doing research on psychotherapy, the review of Smith, Glass, and Miller (1980), in which they performed a metaanalysis on 475 controlled studies of 78 defined psychotherapies, is illuminating. In this study the authors derived 1,766 effect-size measures of psychotherapy. They found that the average person who received psychotherapy was better off at the end of treatment than 80% of those persons with similar symptoms who did not receive treatment. Stated differently, the average person who would score at the fiftieth percentile of the untreated (control) population on measures of emotional well-being could expect to rise to the eightieth percentile of that population after psychotherapy. Their data suggested that the formal psychotherapies are more effective than "undifferentiated counseling." The largest effects appeared to be on measures of subjective emotional experience, such as fear or anxiety, while the smallest seem to be on measures of personality traits and work or school adjustment.

The question of the effectiveness of short-term psychotherapy is an area of special significance to policymakers. Malan (1976) has written on the effectiveness of brief psychoanalytic psychotherapy, using a technique that contains all the essential interpretive elements of full-scale analysis on carefully selected patients. He has argued that this technique results in lasting changes from a relatively brief form of psychotherapy. Other authors have written on the efficacy of different models of short-term psychotherapy (Luborsky et al., 1975; Meltzoff & Kornreich, 1970; Rachman, 1977; Smith et al., 1980). All these authors emphasize the importance of patient selection and maintain that short-term approaches are not universally applicable.

Regarding the effects of therapist training, the Smith, Glass, and Miller review (1980) found that experimenters trained in psychology obtained the largest effects, followed by those trained in psychiatry and education, in that order. These psychologists were most frequently engaged in studies involving behavioral therapies on monophobic clients, while the other groups were treating a wider array of disorders.

Effective psychotherapy, it would appear, may be skillfully provided by welltrained and selected therapists of various mental
health disciplines. Aside from the value of an accurate diagnosis,
however, if psychotherapy alone could cure most patients with
schizophrenia, depression, and the neuroses, why should the
therapist need to go to medical school? By that same token, if
antipsychotics alone cured schizophrenia, antidepressants cured
depression, and anxiolytics cured neuroses, why would one need
a specialist? *It is the ability to integrate these modalities effectively that
makes a psychiatrist the person to treat a significant number of patients
with a mental disorder.*

Cost-Effectiveness

At a time of public and political concern about escalating health
care costs, questions about cost and the feasibility of third-party
coverage for the provisions of mental health services are of critical importance.

First, it is important to acknowledge the rationale for the provision of mental health services, namely, alleviation of the individual's
pain of mental illness, helping the individual and family lead more
productive lives, and the curtailment of a ripple effect of mental
illness in families and larger social units. These goals can be
achieved at reasonable cost, especially when one notes that part of the
expense is offset by savings in other segments of the medical care
system. An "offset effect" occurs when the use of mental health services
leads to a reduction in the use of other health care services. The areas
of overlap in health care delivery for the medical and emotional
aspects of illness are extensive and complex (see Chapter 4).

Of special significance are studies of psychiatric symptoms caused
by previously unrecognized, often subtle, neurological, endocrine,
and other physical illnesses. Some studies estimate that an underlying physical illness is the primary cause of psychiatric symptoms in
approximately 9% to 18% of patients referred or self-referred to a
psychiatrist. This is seen in a variety of physical illnesses including
alcohol and drug abuse; some cancers; certain endocrine, central
nervous system, metabolic, toxic nutritional, and infectious disor-

ders; also in side effects of many prescribed medications. Occasionally, such psychiatric symptoms may preceed by months the physical signs and symptoms of the underlying physical illness. On the other hand, a mental illness may be manifested, initially, by a wide variety of physical complaints. These symptoms may be, diagnostically, not only very challenging, but also may be mislead and may misdirect attention into a fruitless and expensive quest for nonexistent underlying organic reasons for the patient's difficulties. Some examples of the cooccurrence of medical and psychiatric illness are demonstrated by such authors as Kaufman (1959), who found a 67% incidence of emotional problems in medically hospitalized patients, and Nigro (1970), who found that 47% of patients who come to medical hospitalization had mental health problems associated with their medical problems.

Furthermore, much of modern medical treatment, while prolonging life, is associated with serious psychiatric complications. Examples of this are to be found in the high incidence of psychotic reactions following open-heart surgery (Kimball, 1969), the high incidence of depression in intensive care units (Andreasen & Norris, 1972), and a 5% suicide rate (four times the general population rate) among chronic hemodialysis patients (Abram, Moore, & Westervelt, 1971).

Schlesinger, Mumford and Glass (1980) reported that 47% of psychiatric patients have significant medical problems and that the effects of the mental illnesses frequently interfere with their proper medical management.

Most of the "offset" research in the U.S. has been done in prepaid group settings (HMOs). These "closed systems" of health care delivery provide a relatively controlled population sample. Of particular note have been the studies of Follette and Cummings (1967) and Norfleet and Burnell (1981) at Kaiser-Permanente in California; Goldensohn (1977) and Goldensohn and Fink (1979) at HIP in New York; Goldberg, Krantz, and Locke (1970) at the Group Health Association of Washington, D.C.; Kessler, Steinwachs, and Hankin (1982) at the Columbia Medical Plan in Maryland; Anderson (1981) at the Medical Center Health Plan in Minnesota; Schlesinger,

Mumford, and Glass (1980) with the Blue Cross/Blue Shield Plan for Federal Employees as well as an extensive review by Jones and Vischi (1979) at the Alcohol, Drug Abuse, and Mental Health Administration (ADAMHA); and the metaanalysis of Mumford, Schlesinger, Glass, Patrick, and Cuerdon (1984).

These authors have uniformly documented significant offset effects in terms of reduced nonpsychiatric medical utilization when mental health services are provided. The orientation of the mental health programs in these settings tends to focus on short-term, goal-oriented, problem-solving therapies with a limited availability of the more intensive long-term therapies. (Anderson, 1981; Goldensohn, 1977)

Flaws in the offset studies mostly involve methodological limitations, a problem not unexpected in clinical research exploring multivarient, multisystem issues. The major problem in otherwise well-matched control samples is that the control patients have not sought or reached psychiatric treatment. There is, however, one recent study in which this problem is partially met by use of a waiting list population as a control group (Kessler et al., 1982). The results of this study are similar to the others noted. Additionally, in a recent extensive review by Mumford and associates (1984), these authors also found that random-assignment studies had similar though lesser offset effects as compared to studies of self-selected patients (33.1% versus 10.4%). The short time span of one to three years involved in follow-up has also been criticized, although some recent studies have reported on follow-up periods of five to eight years (Follette & Cummings, 1967; White, 1981).

Most studies have not described the specific nature of the psychotherapy provided, although there seems to be a suggested trend that the more "formal" therapies, as opposed to "counseling" or "educational" models, are more effective (Mumford, Schlesinger, & Glass, 1982). Finally, McGuire and Montgomery (1982) have suggested that the potential for offset effects may be less in the fee-for-service sector that in an HMO. In private practice there might be more impetus to treat for optimal psychiatric goals rather than "return-to-function." Even here, however, Jameson, Shuman, and Young

(1978) describe similar trends. This study demonstrated about a 30% reduction in medical utilization associated with psychotherapy provided on a fee-for-service basis. Mumford and others' (1984) recent metaanalysis study has confirmed this offset effect of fee-for-service systems.

Jones and Vischi (1979) found that all 12 studies of alcohol treatment in HMO settings demonstrated an offset effect ranging from 26%-69%, with a median of 40%. They, likewise, found 12 of 13 studies of medical utilization by patients with nonalcohol-related mental illnesses to show offsets ranging from 5%-80%, with a median of 20%. Mumford and others (1984) found that 85% of 65 studies examined demonstrated offset.

Jameson and associates' study (1978) of high medical utilization patients demonstrated an offset, following the initiation of mental health treatment, of 57% in medical and surgical costs and 45% in inpatient psychiatric costs. This was associated with an 80% increase in outpatient psychiatric costs for a net decline of 31% in total costs. The savings from reduced medical-surgical care more than covered the cost of the psychiatric care provided.

Anderson (1981) found that following the institution of integrated mental health services, the admission rate for chemical dependency problems dropped from 2.02 per 1,000 to 0.77 per 1,000, and the hospitalization rate for mental illness decreased from 1.57 to 0.43 per 1,000 population. Mumford and associates' (1984) review of those studies comparing inpatient and outpatient medical utilization, with an average change of 73.4% for inpatient and 22.6% of outpatient usage. Since 75% of health care costs are derived from inpatient expenses, the significance of this trend is obvious.

An important question that arises is how much mental health treatment needs to be provided before these offset benefits are seen. Some studies (Goldberg et al., 1970) have demonstrated a significant offset with only one mental health visit, while others (Kessler et al., 1982; Norfleet & Burnell, 1981) have demonstrated a dose-response relationship. For example, the Kaiser-Permanente studies divided their cohort of referred high medical utilizers into groups of high and low mental health utilizers and found that the high mental health utilizers had a greater diminution in their medical care usage (Follette & Cummings, 1967; Norfleet & Burnell, 1981). The question of whether this is mere substitution of psychiatric overutilization for medical/surgical overutilization has been of concern. The preponderance of the evidence (Follette & Cummings, 1967; Schlesinger, Mumford, Glass, Patrick, & Sharfstein 1983), however, suggests that medical utilization for most patients does not increase after the completion of the course of psychotherapy, especially when short-term therapy models are employed. In fact, one study (Goldberg et al., 1970) reported that even referral for mental health services without actual treatment decreased overall utilization. Rosen and Wiens (1979) agree that even brief contact (one or two visits) has some offset effect.

The majority of studies (Jones and Vischi, 1979; Kessler et al., 1982; Rosen & Wiens, 1979) confirm that psychotherapeutic contact is a significant factor. The Hopkins-based study (Kessler et al., 1982) suggests that the most dramatic offset occurs in patients with moderate use of psychiatric care—in the range of two to 10 visits. On an individual basis, patients who were candidates for brief therapy for conditions of a relatively immediate nature, receiving highly intensive individual therapy, revealed the greatest offset. The researchers found that patients who have chronic mental illness and those needing psychotropic medications have lesser offsets due to their need for continuing management. Also significant, in view of our aging population, is the finding by Mumford and others (1984) that older patients tend to have the greatest offset effects following mental health treatment.

Of special significance are studies that show that the full offset does not occur immediately, but increases with time (Jones & Vischi, 1979; White, 1981). This seems to occur because the treatment population continues to decrease medical utilization, while generally not requiring ongoing psychiatric care, and because virtually all the control groups are found to have a continuing slow rise in utilization with time (Jameson et al., 1978).

There is a growing body of literature on the benefits of providing a mental health opinion regarding patients with clearly defined medical and surgical disorders. In a review of 34 control studies on postsurgical and postmyocardial infarction patients, Mumford and associates (1984) calculated that psychiatric intervention reduced hospitalization by approximately two days. The majority of the interventions were felt by the authors to be modest. They divided the interventions into two broad classes of interaction—psychotherapeutic and educational—and found that while both were effective, the psychotherapeutic were more so, with a combined approach being superior to either alone. They found the largest effects in the areas of cooperation with treatment, speed of recovery, and reduction in posthospital complications.

In a study of offset effects of psychiatric intervention in patients with chronic medical disease, specifically chronic obstructive pulmonary disease, diabetes mellitus, ischemic heart disease, and hypertension, Schlesinger and associates (1983) found that the saving in medical charges over three years in the group having seven to 20 mental health treatment visits was approximately equal in cost to 20 mental health visits.

The weight of evidence strongly suggests that the provision of mental health services, especially in organized health care settings, not only provides a service that is indispensable to the concept of comprehensive health care and the provision of relief from the suffering of mental illness, but also has spillover or offset effects measured in dollars saved. The implication regarding public policy is that adequate mental health benefits should be provided both for obvious humanitarian reasons and because this can be done economically. Addressing the latter factor, McGuire and Montgomery (1982), in a recent review, point out that based on the experience of those states that mandate mental health coverage in all health insurance coverage, the mandate seems to increase the net costs of insurance provision by about one to two dollars per person per year. This is associated with a 10%–20% increase in the number of psychotherapy services provided.

In summary, several points can be emphasized:

1. Health is composed of interdependent physical and emotional components. Most patients who present for health care services lie somewhere along a spectrum between having purely medical or purely psychiatric problems. It is, therefore, unwise and costly to provide medical and psychiatric services in isolation from each other.
2. A wide range of psychiatric treatments for mental illness and the emotional components of physical illness appear to be clinically effective.
3. There should be an increased emphasis on the provision of mental health services to the aged, who are presently significant underutilizers but who demonstrate the greatest offset benefits.
4. The cost of providing such services is predictably modest if reasonable control measures are taken.
5. Mental health care for patients who reflect their emotional conflicts in somatic terms or who have psychiatric complications of physical illness is frequently best provided *in an integrated fashion* within the primary medical care system. The emphasis in such cases should be on the maintenance of the primary care relationship, with the mental health services being provided in the form of either consultation to the primary caregiver or in a conjoint manner.

Epidemiology of Mental Illness

We believe that psychiatric illness is not a "myth." It is real, prevalent, and specific. The bedrock on which mental health public policy decisions regarding manpower ought to be made is the epidemiology of mental illness. If psychiatry is to be seen as a legitimate medical specialty, then one must address the extent to which mental illnesses, with their broad diversity, fit into a medical epidemiology. For the interested reader, a more comprehensive and thoroughly documented version of this epidemiology is available separately. (Shemo, 1982).

Within the U.S. most studies in this field have focused on

generalized psychiatric disability, rather than on the incidence, prevalence, or morbid risk of specific disorders. Challenging problems remain since prognosis and appropriate treatment issues are increasingly dependent on specific diagnosis.

The major studies of the 1950s and 1960s, including the Midtown Manhattan Study conducted by the Cornell group (Srole, Langner, Michael, Opler, & Rennie, 1962), the Stirling County Study of Leighton, Harding, Macklin, Macmillan, and Leighton (1963), and the New Haven study of Hollingshead and Redlich (1958), tended to avoid existing psychiatric nosology in favor of overall mental impairment. They imply a unitary concept of mental illness related to social causation.

Psychiatric epidemiology has been heavily influenced by sociology, anthropology, and other social sciences (Weissman & Klerman, 1978). For example, Faris and Dunham (1967) in the 1930s studied the demographics of the Chicago mental hospitals and found that the highest rates of hospitalization for mental illness occurred in residents of those geographic areas with the greatest social disorganization. Hollingshead and Redlich (1958) also found that their social Class V category showed a prevalence of mental illness at 16 per 1,000 compared to 6 per 1,000 in the Classes I through IV. These findings did not elucidate the cause and effect relationship between sociologic disadvantage and increased incidence of mental illness.

The above studies demonstrated a degree of prevalence of psychiatric impairment in the community that had not previously been fully appreciated. For example, the Midtown Manhattan Study demonstrated that 23% of the population was substantially impaired and only 19% of the subjects were free of any significant psychiatric symptoms (Srole et al., 1962). Regier, Goldberg, and Taube (1978) at NIMH recently reported a more conservative estimate of 15% of the base population of the U.S. as having significant mental illness.

Another finding of these broad, early studies was that a mental health specialist was not treating the majority of persons with psychiatric disability. Srole and others (1962), for example, demonstrated that only 1 in 20 of those classified as impaired were in treatment. Likewise, Shepherd, Cooper, Brown, and Kalton's (1966) United Kingdom study demonstrated that only 5% of persons with recognizable mental illness were being seen by a psychiatrist.

Of related interest, Tischler, Henisz, Myers, and Boswell's (1975) study of the utilization of mental health services demonstrated that certain groups, such as children and the aged, were significant underutilizers of mental health services as their rates of impairment were far greater than their rates of service utilization.

Several European studies, based on an adherence to Kraepelin's principles, did attempt to document the lifetime prevalence rates for specific diagnostic categories. For example, the post-World War II survey of Lundby, Sweden, conducted by Essen-Moller (Gruenberg, 1980), revealed the prevalence rates indicated in Table 6.1.

Major advances in the basic sciences have led to a renewed appreciation for the heterogeneity of psychiatric disorders and the fact that they have different clinical pictures, natural histories, family aggregations, and responses to treatment (Guze, 1970). Advances in treatment that have evolved from studies using well-delineated diagnostic groups have reinforced a renewed focus on nosology.

Of considerable interest in this regard are the recently published preliminary findings of the NIMH Epidemiological Catchment Area Program (ECA) (Eaton et al., 1984; Myers et al., 1984; Regier et al., 1984; Robins et al., 1984; Shapiro et al., 1984). This study, which involves 20,000 community residents in five states across the U.S., uses an extensive diagnostic interview instrument in an attempt to

Table 6.1
Lifetime Prevalence Rates per 1000 Population

Psychosis	19.5	Schizophrenia	7.0
Affective Psychosis	10.2	Neurosis	58.5
Personality Disorders			
major	64.0	Mental Retardation	9.8
minor	210.0		

arrive at 15 DSM-III diagnoses, rather than measuring only levels of global impairment. Significantly, the study will involve five times the number of subjects than in any prior survey. It involves a one-year follow-up reinterview and contains elaborate precautions to avoid the overcounting of mild or uncertain cases. Its specific goals include the following: 1) an estimation of the rates of prevalence and incidence of specific mental disorders; 2) an estimate of the rates of health and mental health service usage; 3) a study of the factors influencing the development and continuation of disorders; and 4) a study of the factors influencing the use of services. At present, only the initial findings from three sites (New Haven, Connecticut, Baltimore, Maryland, and St. Louis, Missouri), have been tabulated.

Nonetheless, several interesting observations have been made. For example, 28–38% of the population examined in these sites have one of the 15 disorders surveyed. While past studies have implied that the rates of psychiatric impairment are greater for women than for men, this study demonstrates that the rates are approximately equal. The men had greater incidences of alcohol and drug abuse/dependence and antisocial personality disorder, while the women had higher rates of major depression, agoraphobia, and simple phobia. Further, persons in the 24-44 year age-group have the highest rates for all disorders, except for those involving cognitive impairment, with other disorders being approximately twice as prevalent in those younger than age 45. There was little difference in rates between the races. Not unexpectedly, persons with higher education levels had lower rates than residents of inner-city environments.

While the number of studies using discrete psychiatric disorders as dependent variables are small, they suggest the findings presented below.

Organic Brain Syndromes: Delirium

Lipowski (1980) estimated that 5%-15% of all patients on medical and surgical wards of general hospitals present with or develop a delirium. Titchener and associates (1956) found that 7%–8% of random surgical patients had a delirium at some time during their hospitalization. The incidence of delirium in a surgical intensive care unit ranged from 18%–30% and in cardiac care units, up to 20%. Approximately 30% of patients with open-heart surgery were also delirious. Delirium and confusional states are more the rule than the exception on inpatient geriatric units (Bedford, 1959).

Organic Brain Syndromes: Dementia

Wells (1978) estimated that approximately one million Americans over the age of 65 (approximately 5%) have severe dementing disorders, about 65% of these being of the Alzheimer's type. Other dementing disorders occur as sequelae to head trauma, chronic alcoholism, multiple cerebral infarction, and reneal or hepatic failure. The ECA study (Robins et al., 1984) demonstrated severe cognitive impairment in 1.0%–1.3% of adults, with the prevalence increasing linearly with age. This study did not differentiate between delirium and dementia.

Schizophrenia

There are an estimated two million Americans who suffer from schizophrenia, with the risk of developing this disorder between the ages of 15 and 45 being approximately 1% (Kolb & Brodie, 1982). With the use of DSM-III diagnostic criteria and the elimination of schizophreniform disorders, the prevalence of this disorder will most likely drop in newer studies by 20%–30%. Because of the severity of this disorder, the schizophrenic population represents 35.7% of all persons hospitalized in the U.S. The ECA study (Robins et al., 1984) found a prevalence of 1.1%–2.0% in this category.

Affective Illness: Unipolar

This group represents 30%–40% of all psychiatric admissions. Berger estimates that there are 1.5 million episodes of depression treated each year in the U.S., with 4.5–7.5 million episodes going untreated (Berger, 1978). An NIMH study (Kolb & Brodie, 1982) reports that 15% of adults between the ages of 18 and 74 suffer depressive symptoms in any given year, with less than 5% of these persons receiving treatment. The ECA study (Robins et al., 1984) found a prevalence rate of 3.1%–6.7%.

Affective Illness: Bipolar

In the U.S. the occurrence of schizophrenia has likely been over-diagnosed and bipolar affective illness underdiagnosed (Pope & Lipinski, 1978). The admission rate for bipolar illness in the United Kingdom has, until recently, been approximately 18 times greater than that in the U.S. (Kolb & Brodie, 1982). Using the diagnostic criteria available in 1978, Berger estimated incidence of bipolar illness to be 0.3%, which translates into 600,000 treated episodes per year. The ECA study (Robins et al., 1984) found a lifetime prevalence of 0.6%–1.1% for mania but does not attempt to distinguish between bipolar and unipolar depression.

Affective Illness: Dysthymic Disorder

In 1977 Hornstra and Klarsen estimated minor or characterologic depressions to have a one-year prevalence of 47–105 per 100,000, while Barrett, Hurst, DiScala, and Rose (1978) estimated the prevalence at 60 per 1,000.

Phobic and Obsessive-Compulsive Disorders

Gruenberg estimated the prevalence of serious phobic disorders at approximately 1% of the population. This percentage may increase with the recently emerging understanding of the diversity of agoraphobic presentations. He estimated the prevalence of incapacitating obsessive-compulsive disorders at 0.05% of the population (Gruenberg, 1980). The ECA study (Robins et al., 1984) has demonstrated a lifetime prevalence for phobic disorders of 7.8%–23.3%, but the upper-range figure, derived from Baltimore, is markedly discordant with the other sites and will require an explanation. Additionally, panic disorder rates were 1.4%–1.5%, and obsessive-compulsive disorders range from 1.9%–3.0%.

Post-Traumatic Stress Disorders

Helzer, Robins, and Davis (1976) estimated that 26% of Vietnam veterans had "some" psychiatric symptoms, with 7% displaying a full depressive syndrome. Titchener and Kapp (1976) reported that 8% of the survivors of the Buffalo Creek disaster developed incapacitating post-traumatic stress disorders, and Adler (1943) demonstrated such symptomatology in 57% of survivors of the Coconut Grove disaster in one year of follow-up. The ECA study did not include this category.

Personality Disorders

Leighton and associates (1963) estimated that 18% of men and 11% of women present with significant symptoms of character disorder and that the incidence of borderline character disorderlike states was 1.7%. Others suggest that if the broad concept of borderline personality organization as advocated by Kernberg was used, approximately 15% of the population would meet the criteria (Stone, 1981). The ECA study (Robins et al., 1984) surveyed only for antisocial personality disorder and found a lifetime prevalence of 2.1%–3.3%.

Alcohol and Drug Abuse

Selzer (1980) reported that approximately nine million Americans suffer from adverse affects of alcohol abuse, approximately 10% of men and 2%–3% of women (Jones & Vischi, 1979). In 1977 Hunt estimated that there were 3,700,000 or more heroin users in the

United States. The ECA study (Robins et al., 1984) found a lifetime prevalence of 1.5%–15.7% for alcohol abuse/dependence and 5.5%–5.8% for drug abuse/dependence.

Summary

While the above figures are derived from, at times, widely varying or poorly specified population samples, they do confirm the impression that the prevalence of psychiatric disorders in the population is substantial. Further, it is possible to distinguish specific diagnostic entities that have some relationship to incidence, prognosis, and treatment. Manpower needs in the mental health field would seem to be reasonably determined by two factors: 1) the prevalence and incidence of specific disorders; and 2) the expertise needed to treat these specific conditions.

References

Abram, H., Moore, G., & Westervelt, F. Suicidal behavior in chronic dialysis patients. *American Journal of Psychiatry*, 127:1199–1204, 1971.

Adler, A. Neuropsychiatric complications in victims of Boston's coconut grove disaster. *Journal of the American Medical Association*, 123:1098, 1943.

Anderson, R. Shifting from external to internal provision of mental health services in a health maintenance organization. *Hospital & Community Psychiatry*, 32(5):311–319, 1981.

Andreasen, N., & Norris, A. Long-term adjustment and adaptation mechanisms in severely burned adults. *Journal of Nervous and Mental Disease*, 154:352–362, 1972.

Barrett, J., Hurst, M., DiScala, C., & Rose, R. Prevalence of depression over a 12-month period in a non-patient population. *Archives of General Psychiatry*, 35:741, 1978.

Bedford, P. General medical aspects of confusional states in elderly people. *British Medical Journal*, 5145:185–188, 1959.

Berger, P. Medical treatment of mental illness. *Science*, 200:974, 1978.

Bergin, A.E. The evaluation of therapeutic outcomes. In A.E. Bergin & S.L. Garfield (Eds.), *Handbook of Psychotherapy and Behavior Change*. New York: Wiley, 1971.

Davis, J.M. Overview: Maintenance therapy in psychiatry: II. Affective disorders. *American Journal of Psychiatry*, 133:1–13, 1976.

Davis, J.M., Shaffer, C.B., Killian, G.A., Kinard, C., and Chan, C. Important issues in the drug treatment of schizophrenia, *Schizophrenia Bulletin*, 6:70–87, 1980.

Eaton, W., Holzer, C., III, Von Korff, M., Anthony, J., Helzer, J., George, L.,

Burnam, A., Boyd, J., Kessler, L., & Locke, B. The design of the epidemiologic catchment area surveys. *Archives of General Psychiatry*, 41:942–948, 1984.

Epstein, N.B., & Vlok, L.A. Research on the results of psychotherapy: A summary of evidence. *American Journal of Psychiatry*, 138:1027–1035, 1981.

Eysenck, H.J. *The Effects of Psychotherapy*. New York: International Science Press, 1966.

Faris, R., & Dunham, H. *Mental Disorders in Urban Areas: An Ecological Study of Schizophrenia and Other Psychosis*. Chicago: The University of Chicago Press, 1967.

Follette, W., & Cummings, N. Psychiatric services and medical utilization in a prepaid health plan setting. *Medical Care*, 5(1):25–35, 1967.

Goldberg, I., Krantz, G., & Locke, B. Effect of a short-term outpatient psychiatric therapy benefit in the utilization of medical services in a prepaid group practice medical program. *Medical Care*, 8(5):419–428, 1970.

Goldensohn, S., & Fink, R. Mental health services for medicaid enrollees in a prepaid group practice plan. *American Journal of Psychiatry*, 136(2):160–164, 1979.

Goldensohn, S. Cost, utilization and utilization review of mental health services in a prepaid group practice plan. *American Journal of Psychiatry*, 134(11):1222–1226, 1977.

Gruenberg, E. Epidemiology. In H. Kaplan, A. Freedman, & B. Saddock (Eds.), *Comprehensive Textbook of Psychiatry/III* (pp. 531–548). Baltimore: Williams & Wilkins, 1980.

Guze, S. The need for toughmindedness in psychiatric thinking. *Southern Medical Journal*, 63:662–671, 1970.

Helzer, J., Robins, L., & Davis, D. Depressive disorders in Vietnam veterans returning. *Journal of Nervous and Mental Disease*, 163:177, 1976.

Hollingshead, A., & Redlich, F. *Social Class and Mental Illness*. New York: John Wiley & Sons, 1958.

Hornstra, R., & Klarsen, D. The course of depression. *Comprehensive Psychiatry*, 18:119, 1977.

Hunt, L.G. Prevalence of active heroin use in the United States. In J.D. Rittenhouse (Ed.), *The Epidemiology of Heroin and Other Narcotics* (p. 61). (NIDA Research Monograph No. 16). Washington, DC: U.S. Government Printing Office, 1977.

Jameson, J., Shuman, L., & Young, W. The effects of outpatient utilization on the costs of providing third-party coverage. *Medical Care*, 16:383–397, 1978.

Jones, K., & Vischi, LT. Impact of alcohol drug abuse and mental health treatment on medical care utilization [supplement]. *Medical Care*, 17(12):1–82, 1979.

Kaufman, M. Psychiatric findings on admission to a medical service in a general hospital. *Journal of the Mount Sinai Hospital*, 26:160–170, 1959.

Kessler, L., Steinwachs, D., & Hankin, J. Episodes of psychiatric care and medical utilization. *Medical Care*, 20(12):1209–1221, 1982.

Kimball, C. Psychological responses to the experience of open-heart surgery: I. *American Journal of Psychiatry*, 126:348–349, 1969.

Klein, D.F., & Davis, J.M. *Diagnosis and Drug Treatment of Psychiatric Disorders*. Baltimore: Williams & Wilkins, 1969.

Klein, D.F., Gittleman, R., Quitkin, F., & Rifkin, A. *Diagnosis and Drug Treatment of*

Psychiatric Disorders: Adults and Children (2nd ed.). Baltimore: Williams & Wilkins, 1980.

Kolb, L., & Brodie, H. *Modern Clinical Psychiatry.* Philadelphia: W.B. Saunders Co., 1982.

Leighton, D., Harding, J., Macklin, D., Macmillan, A., & Leighton, A. *The Character of Danger, Volume 3, The Stirling County Study of Psychiatric Disorder and Sociocultural Environment.* New York: Basic Books, 1963.

Lipowski, Z. Organic mental disorders: Introduction and review of syndromes. In H. Kaplan, A. Freedman, & B. Saddock (Eds.), *Comprehensive Textbook of Psychiatry/III* (pp. 1359–1392). Baltimore: Williams & Wilkins, 1980.

Luborsky, L., Singer, B., & Luborsky, L. Comparative studies of psychotherapies. *Archives of General Psychiatry,* 32:995–1008, 1975.

Malan, D.H. *The Frontier of Brief Psychotherapy: An Example of the Convergence of Research and Clinical Practice.* New York and London: Plenum Medical Book Co., 1976.

McGuire, T. & Montgomery, F. Mandated mental health benefits in private health insurance. *Journal of Health Politics and Law,* 7(2):380–406, 1982.

Meltzoff, J., & Kornreich, M. *Research in Psychotherapy.* Chicago: Aldine, 1970.

Mumford, E., Schlesinger, H., Glass, G., Patrick, C., & Cuerdon, T. A new look at evidence about reduced cost of medical utilizations following mental health treatment. *American Journal of Psychiatry,* 141:1145–1158, 1984.

Mumford, E., Schlesinger, H., & Glass, G. The effects of psychological intervention on recovery from surgery and heart attacks: An analysis of the literature. *American Journal of Public Health,* 72(2):141–151, 1982.

Myers, J., Weissman, M., Tischler, G., Holzer, C., III, Leaf, P., Orvaschel, H., Anthony, J., Boyd, J., Burke, J., Jr., Kramer, M., & Stoltzmanl, R. Six-month prevalence of psychiatric disorders in three communities. *Archives of General Psychiatry,* 41:959–967, 1984.

Nigro, S.A. Psychiatrists' experiences in general practice in a hospital emergency room. *Journal of the American Medical Association,* 214:1657–1660, 1970.

Norfleet, M., & Burnell, G. Utilization of medical services by psychiatric patients. *Hospital & Community Psychiatry,* 32(3):198–200, 1981.

Pope, H., & Lipinski, J. Diagnosis in schizophrenia and manic depressive illness. *Archives of General Psychiatry,* 35:811–828, 1978.

Rachman, S. Double standards and single standards. *Bulletin of the British Psychological Society,* 30:295, 1977.

Regier, D., Goldberg, I., & Taube, C. The de facto U.S. mental health services system: A public health perspective. *Archives of General Psychiatry,* 35:685–693, 1978.

Regier, D., Myers, J., Kramer, M., Robins, L., Blazer, D., Hough, R., Eaton, W., & Locke, B. The NIMH epidemiologic catchment area program. *Archives of General Psychiatry,* 41:934–941, 1984.

Robins, L., Helzer, J., Weissman, M., Orvaschel, H., Gruenberg, E., Burke J., Jr. & Regier, D. Lifetime prevalence of specific psychiatric disorders in three sites. *Archives of General Psychiatry,* 41:949–958, 1984.

Rosen, J., & Wiens, A. Changes in medical problems and use of medical services following psychological intervention. *American Psychologist,* 34(5):420–431, 1979.

Schlesinger, H., Mumford, E., Glass, G., Patrick, C., & Sharfstein, S. Mental health treatment and medical care utilization in a fee-for-service system: Outpatient mental health treatment following the onset of chronic disease. *American Journal of Public Health,* 73(4):422–429, 1983.

Schlesinger, H., Mumford, E., & Glass, G. Mental health services and medical utilization. In G. Vandenbos (Ed.), *Psychotherapy Practice, Research, Policy.* Beverly Hills: Sage, 1980.

Selzer, M. Alcoholism and alcoholic psychosis. In H. Kaplan, A. Freedman, & B. Saddock (Eds.), *Comprehensive Textbook of Psychiatry/III* (pp. 1629–1645). Baltimore: Williams & Wilkins, 1980.

Shapiro, S., Skinner, E., Kessler, L., Von Korff, M., German, P., Tischler, G., Leaf, P., Benhan, L., Cottler, L., & Regier, D. Utilization of health and mental health services. *Archives of General Psychiatry,* 41:971–978, 1984.

Shemo, J. *New epidemiology of mental illnesses.* Unpublished report, University of Virginia School of Medicine, Charlottesville, VA, 1982.

Shepherd, M., Cooper, B., Brown, A., & Kalton, G. *Psychiatric Illness in General Practice.* London: Oxford University Press, 1966.

Smith, M.L., Glass, G.V., & Miller, T.I. *The Benefits of Psychotherapy.* Baltimore & London: The Johns Hopkins University Press, 1980.

Srole, L., Langner, T., Michael, S., Opler, M., & Rennie, T. *Mental Health in the Metropolis: The Midtown Manhattan Study.* New York: McGraw-Hill, 1962.

Stone, M. Borderline syndromes. A consideration of subtypes and an overview, directions for research. *Psychiatric Clinics of North America,* 4:1, 1981.

Tischler, G., Henisz, J., Myers, J., & Boswell, P. Utilization of mental health services: I. Patienthood and the prevalence of symptomatology in the community. *Archives of General Psychiatry,* 32:411–418, 1975.

Titchener, E., & Kapp, F. Family and character change at Buffalo Creek. *American Journal of Psychiatry,* 133:295, 1976.

Titchener, J., Zwerling, I., Gottschalk, L., Levine, M., Sulvertson, W., Cohen, S., & Silver, H. Psychosis in surgical patients. *Surgery, Gynecology & Obstetrics,* 102:59, 1956.

Weissman, M., & Klerman, G. Epidemiology of mental disorders: Emerging trends in the United States. *Archives of General Psychiatry,* 35:705–712, 1978.

Wells, C. Chronic brain disease: An overview. *American Journal of Psychiatry,* 135:1–12, 1978.

White, S. The impact of mental health services on medical care utilization: Economic and organizational implications. *Hospital & Community Psychiatry,* 32(5):311–319, 1981.

7

ROLES FOR TOMORROW'S PSYCHIATRIST

Before suggesting directions for the future, we will first restate the major problems facing today's mentally ill (Chapter 2) and then recommend changes in the roles of psychiatrists that would seem to address these issues. We will not suggest possible new roles for other mental health disciplines.

Major Problem Areas

While our society today has achieved considerable success in prolonging life, reducing suffering, and improving the functioning of many of the mentally ill, three remaining problems stand out:

1. our society's abrogation of responsibility for the treatment of tens of thousands of people with severe psychiatric illness who now roam the nation's city streets;
2. the lack of access to effective treatment for many patients who see a variety of therapists or primary-care physicians whose knowledge is less than comprehensive;
3. the increasing presence of economic barriers to psychiatric treatment for all but the affluent.

Mentally Ill Who Are Not in Treatment

Over the past quarter of a century, a national policy of deinstitutionalization has resulted in a public abandonment of responsibility for many citizens with chronic, disabling mental illness. We face a growing mental health crisis as the number of mentally ill who are homeless, living in the streets, and receiving no psychiatric treatment increases. Other mentally ill patients, assigned to "back ward" board and care homes, or residing in local jails, may receive fragmented social services, but they have no one available who is *responsible* for providing their psychiatric treatment. These persons, most of whom are affected by severe, chronic mental illnesses, should have access to a professional responsible for creating and maintaining a physician-patient relationship in order to address their needs. Such a relationship is traditionally characterized by mutual trust and an uncompromising concern about obtaining the best treatment for the patient. Stated differently, these patients cannot cope with both a devastating mental illness and the normal demands of modern urban society without help from someone trained in the role of being responsible for patients. "Providers," defined as persons who supply a service, or even "case managers," who are supposed to coordinate a variety of providers' services, are an inadequate substitute for the physician-patient relationship. While addressing their *treatment* needs, these seriously disabled people should be considered "patients," not primarily "clients," "consumers," "customers," "cases," "recipients," "subjects," or "students."

Patients with a major mental illness require someone with a combination of orientations to treat them. For example, even those who respond quite well to psychotropic medications, very often need psychological and social approaches to achieve compliance with treatment. Of the mental health disciplines, the psychiatrist is least wedded to a single science or point of view. Psychiatrists who are not committed to a single treatment modality can choose among or combine approaches from a range of knowledge, depending on the needs of each patient. *Patients with a serious mental illness will be helped by standards that require psychiatrists to provide or direct the provision of combined treatment approaches.*

Patients with a chronic mental illness often need the skills of different disciplines, including psychiatrists and other physicians, psychologists, social workers, nurses, ministers, adjunctive therapists, and a variety of counselors. These patients often can use the skills of a multidisciplinary team even more than those with less severe, better understood, or more easily treated illnesses. In addition to the basic caring attitude expected from any discipline, these patients additionally often need the intimate "hands-on" care traditionally provided by nurses. They generally require the specific skills in environmental structuring known to social workers. Like a good football team, a treatment team needs members who offer a variety of specific skills in addition to their overall knowledge of the game. Moreover, these various skills are best melded under a leadership that assumes responsibility for the whole patient and is trained to combine a variety of orientations.

Inadequate Access to Effective Treatment

As Chapter 4 on the primary care system points out, many patients with diagnosed (and undiagnosed) mental illness are receiving less than optimum treatment in that system. Earlier chapters also suggest a similar inadequacy in community mental health programs due to deprofessionalization of their staffs. A scrutiny of much of the current work of all the mental health disciplines would likely disclose a similar lack of diagnostic precision and comprehensive treatment. Clinicians skilled in psychiatric examination and diagnosis who can provide a sense of medical responsibility and a breadth of conception are needed not only to provide treatment of major mental disorders, but also to address the needs of patients with other illnesses such as affective and somatization disorders, anxiety disorders, and certain character disorders, as well as the complex disorders of childhood and the elderly. This need is particularly pressing in the initial evaluation and treatment planning, where the integration of knowledge from a number of sciences is so valuable. *We recommend, therefore, that persons with psychiatric illnesses enter the health care system at points where such comprehensive diagnosing and treatment planning are available.*

Economic Barriers

A third major issue is that of inadequate insurance coverage for the mentally ill. Virtually all health insurance, including Medicare and Medicaid, discriminate against patients with mental or emotional illness. If mental health insurance expenses could be limited to the treatment of bona fide mental illness, perhaps the insuring institutions would be more willing to remedy this inequity. There are at least three conceptual boundaries that create difficulties: 1) distinguishing "patients with illnesses" from "clients with problems in living"; 2) distinguishing these "patients" from welfare recipients with social needs; and 3) distinguishing "patients with illnesses" from "students" with educational needs. Some of the "personal growth" or "training" therapies may fall into the third category. In addition to the burden of their illnesses, many of the mentally ill have severe problems in living, social deficits, and educational and vocational needs that may have to be addressed by combinations of funding from sources other than health dollars alone.

In the development and revision of the third edition of the *Diagnostic and Statistical Manual for Mental Disorders* (APA, 1980), the American Psychiatric Association has made considerable progress in delimiting diagnostic boundaries. As the psychiatric profession sharpens its definition of "illness," the rationale for equivalent health insurance coverage should improve. Moreover, to the extent that psychiatrists are perceived as treating patients with illnesses rather than as solving "normal" problems in living, our society will recognize that psychiatrists are physicians and that their patients should have the same access to health insurance as people with physical illnesses.

Professional Standards for Psychiatrists

As one reads the chapters in the appendix on psychology, social work, and nursing, it is apparent that each discipline regards its members as independent agents in the treatment of mental disorders. Had we extended our appendix to include descriptions of pastoral counselors, marriage counselors, substance abuse counselors, occupational therapists, and so on, we could also obtain additional calls from those disciplines for greater professional autonomy. Psychiatrists cannot speak for any of the other disciplines as to their professional identities or aspirations. We do, however, feel a responsibility to describe our views about psychiatry in terms of that which best serves psychiatric patients. In discussing the future roles of psychiatrists, we will first address professional standards, then discuss implications for training, research, and public policy.

In Chapter 3 we propose that psychiatry is a specialty of medicine with three unique characteristics: 1) the tradition of responsibility for the mentally ill within a physician-patient relationship (the therapeutic alliance); 2) the ability to perform comprehensive diagnostic assessments; and 3) the ability to integrate knowledge from a wide range of sciences and theories in determining the most effective treatment approach. We note that the enormous growth of knowledge in mental health fields (cf. Chapter 6) has made it difficult for many psychiatrists to attain expertise in all areas. Consequently, a good number have tended to specialize. Psychoanalysts and some dynamic psychotherapists, for example, have spent a protracted postresidency training for mastery of those techniques. Other psychiatrists have focused upon biological research or upon prevention of mental illness through social interventions.

If specialization focuses upon specific illnesses, restricted age groups, or practice in specific settings, a psychiatrist can retain a broad medical perspective in applying the three unique characteristics even though his or her focus is narrowed. However, by specializing in techniques such as hypnosis, family psychotherapy, psychoanalysis, or psychopharmacology, the psychiatrist's orientation to patients may tend to change from that of a traditional physician-patient relationship, in which the broad range of diagnostic and therapeutic techniques are available, to that of a provider of a specific service. In other words, the psychiatric subspecialist, whose focus is only on technique, may lose the perspective of a broad-based clinician and, in determining the diagnosis of a patient's illness, may tend to formulate the problem only in terms of the theory underlying his or her technique. Of course a psychiatrist may become expert at a specific technique and, *in addition*, retain the three unique characteristics of psychiatry.

Furthermore, funders, educators, and even some professionals have difficulty understanding the differences between a psychiatrist performing social or psychological techniques and other well-trained mental health professionals performing the same techniques. This focus on technique rather than professional background tends to blur professional differences rather than clarify them, a situation that tends to confuse potential patients and referral sources alike. *We therefore contend that psychiatric patients will be better served if psychiatrists retain their identity as physicians, including the three unique characteristics described above, rather than risk blurring their professional identity with that of other mental health professionals by focusing only on techniques.*

Primary and Subspecialized Psychiatrists

Organized psychiatry should evolve a process for identifying those psychiatrists who have retained the capacity and interest to perform the basic psychiatric skills described above. For want of a better term, we might call them "primary psychiatrists." Others who choose to limit themselves to providing a specialized skill, task, or service we might call "subspecialized psychiatrists." Because these subspecialists have honed a given skill to an exceptionally competent level, they will remain essential in providing treatment for many patients with complex psychiatric illnesses. Moreover, many psychiatrists are capable of maintaining both the primary and subspecialist roles, as frequently occurs within other medical disciplines.

Conceptually, those physicians who are to be regarded as primary psychiatrists should be capable of the following:

1. establishing physician-patient relationships and assuming medical responsibility for patients entering into psychiatric treatment;
2. performing thorough psychiatric examinations and diagnostic assessments, that is, identifying the disorder, ruling out other possible disorders, and formulating the social, psychological, and biological factors contributing to the illness; and

3. determining the most effective and efficient comprehensive treatments for each patient and either treating the patient or making appropriate referrals.

Consistent with this concept, *psychiatric standards should require that any patient with a mental illness have an initial evaluation by a primary psychiatrist in order to determine the diagnosis and treatment needs.* The primary psychiatrist may treat or refer patients to subspecialists or other mental health practitioners depending on the needs of the patient and the knowledge and interest of the psychiatrist. Psychiatric subspecialists who have not maintained their primary psychiatric skills should treat patients with mental illness only upon referral from primary psychiatrists. A psychopharmacologist or psychoanalyst, however, who has retained the unique skills of psychiatry is in a position to be both a primary psychiatrist and subspecialized psychiatrist. Moreover, this concept does not preclude subspecialists (or any other mental health professional, for that matter) from providing their services to "clients," or educating "students," if they wish.

Over time, certification by the American Board of Psychiatry and Neurology could be seen as designating who is a primary psychiatrist. To do so immediately would not be practical because a large number of very capable psychiatrists are currently not board certified. Nonetheless, certification of primary psychiatrists should be considered a long-range goal of the profession. Moreover, the profession may wish to encourage subspecialization certification over time—for example, in geropsychiatry or substance abuse. By increasing the meaning of certification, psychiatry can increase the public trust in the profession.

This proposal does not imply that psychiatrists should provide treatment for all mentally ill patients. In addition to making referrals to psychiatric subspecialists, the primary psychiatrist might make independent referrals to other medical or mental health disciplines. For example, a primary psychiatrist who does not treat phobias might refer a phobic patient to a psychologist who specializes in such disorders, with the understanding that the patient need not return unless the treatment fails. A psychiatrist who is not skilled in family therapy may refer the family of an alcoholic patient, whose behavior is causing family disruption, to a social worker specializing in the treatment of alcohol abuse and family therapy. A psychiatrist may see a chronic schizophrenic patient at spaced intervals to assess the patient's condition, evaluate his need for medications, and review the treatment plan in collaboration with a psychiatric nurse/clinician who performs psychiatric nursing assessments and provides family counseling and health education on bimonthly home visits. Similarly, a patient with diabetes, hypertension, and a stabilized affective disorder may be referred to an internist for ongoing medical treatment, with the understanding that the psychiatrist be called in consultation if the patient becomes unstable emotionally.

This proposal may sound quixotic today to our most politically pragmatic psychiatrists, while sounding unnecessarily restrictive to the many psychiatrists who effectively and efficiently treat a broad variety of psychiatric illnesses. However, we can most surely predict that in the future *the knowledge in psychiatry required to practice effectively will continue to grow.* This expansion of knowledge will no doubt increase the diversity and the complexity of psychiatry. *The question before American psychiatry is not whether subspecialization will occur, but what form it will take.* Allowing such specialization to evolve as a function of self-starting groups will produce a hodgepodge of subspecialization that will leave patients confused about who is to serve whom, leave the public confused as to who speaks to what problem, and leave the profession highly disorganized and probably highly conflictual. *Thus psychiatry needs an organizational concept of subspecialization to provide a framework to approach this complexity and to create credible standards.*

How do we envision the typical psychiatrist of 2000 A.D.? An example might help. The psychiatrist (in our example, a woman) will have a sense of broad medical responsibility for patients coming to her, as well as skills in evaluating the psychiatric needs of her patients. In addition to these primary skills, she will have specialized in a major diagnostic entity, for instance, affective illnesses (we could have selected an age group or another diagnostic grouping). She will retain responsibility for patients within her areas of expertise, including those with affective disorders, but will refer patients who need specialized skills outside of her competence. One might visualize her knowledge as shaped like a "T," with broad evaluation skills for all mental disorders, but in-depth knowledge and skills primarily for one disorder (see Figure 7.1).

Being responsible for affective disorders will require constant enhancement of her interpersonal, intrapsychic, neurochemical, neurophysiological, psychopharmacological, genetic, and familial knowledge of the illnesses, and ongoing enhancement of her psychotherapeutic and psychopharmacological skills relative to affective disorders. She will be current in knowledge and skills needed to provide a comprehensive range of possible treatments for affective disorders. Moreover, she will maintain her facility in the comprehensive diagnosis and treatment of patients with multiple disorders, such as a combination of affective disorder and alcoholism.

In addition, she will stay current in those general skills that entitle her to be a primary psychiatrist. Sometimes, despite her in-depth knowledge, she will find situations in the treatment of her patients that she believes should be addressed by referral or collab-

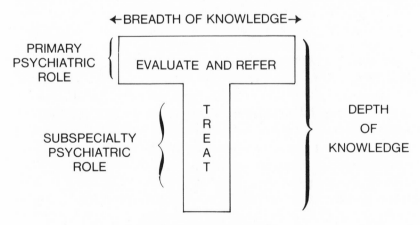

Figure 7.1. T-Diagram

oration. For instance, she may have a patient with a bipolar illness whose complex family relationships seem to precipitate an exacerbation of symptoms. If she has not developed her skills in family therapy to the extent that she can address the family constellations, or she prefers to maintain an individual relationship with her patient, she may refer such a patient to a psychiatrist (or other mental health professional) who she knows is skilled in such therapy. She will retain overall responsibility for the patient and will maintain periodic communication with the family therapist regarding the patient's progress. She may also refer patients who do not have an affective disorder to other professionals.

An analogy is seen in internal medicine today. Internists have refined their skills as we have outlined, and some have specialized in a group of diseases. Often they will refer, or not accept, patients other than those about whom they have a subspecialized knowledge.

We are not suggesting that individual practitioners will not have varying professional identities. For instance, a psychiatrist may maintain primary skills, have in-depth understanding of a category of illnesses, and accept referrals for specific procedures, such as group or family psychotherapy. Our major theme is that regardless of these complexities, each patient will first have a relationship with a primary psychiatrist. If highly specialized skills are required, the patient may also have a relationship with a subspecialist—who, of course, may also be the primary psychiatrist.

Psychiatric Medicine

We do not foresee psychiatry moving toward a more biological, more psychosocial, or more psychodynamic perspective. Instead, we see the profession identifying with the *integration* of all those areas within a medical perspective. By "medical" we mean that combination of art, science, and humanity that has guided physicians in treating patients for centuries. *In no sense do we limit "medicine" to its "biological" dimension.* We have searched the contributions of other professions involved with mental illness. We find no other discipline with the necessary background (or inclination) to "treat the whole patient"—mind and body in a social context. We do not see the field merging with other medical specialties, such as internal medicine or neurology, because to do so would leave patients without a physician willing and able to provide our unique integrative function of mind, body, and behavior in a social context.

No one else has the background to integrate biological, social, and psychological aspects of human behavior from a medical frame of reference. Psychiatric medicine has been, is, and will continue to be a unique, diverse, professional field that is sorely needed by our society and should remain economically rewarding. Psychiatrists offer a wide array of skills and knowledge that no other profession or medical specialty can match, and our knowledge base is growing with every publication.

The Clinical Team

This proposal conceptualizes the mental health team often found in organized settings as embracing diverse skills. A variety of skills is particularly useful where difficult, chronic, or refractory patients need multidisciplinary approaches. Alternatively, when knowledge regarding accurate diagnosis permits a single specific treatment approach, the multidisciplinary team approach is unnecessary and wasteful. In order to conserve resources, such a team approach should be assigned only to those patients who meet established criteria for difficulty or complexity. Teams should include a primary psychiatrist who can establish a physician-patient relationship and who accepts responsibility for overall care, makes the diagnosis (or diagnoses), and plays a major role in the combined treatment planning that these refractory patients need. A clinical team should consist of specialists, each of whom has clear-cut clinical skills that, in toto, provide the patient with the services required.

Disabled persons who have a chronic paranoid schizophrenic illness, for example, need the highly developed diagnostic and treatment planning skills of a psychiatrist within a responsible and supportive physician-patient relationship. In addition, they often need environmental structuring, help with financial problems, help with unrealistic family expectations, behavioral techniques or psychodrama, group or individual psychotherapy, counseling, resocialization, or help from the various occupational, vocational, or recreational therapies. Some of these skills may be provided by social workers, nurses, psychologists, or specific adjunctive therapists at various levels of training. Just as football teams use specialists in punting, running, tackling or catching passes, clinical teams need members with in-depth skills in specific areas in order to provide the patient with the breadth of skilled therapeutic tasks that are needed. A football team will do poorly if everyone insists on being the pass receiver; patients with severe mental illness are poorly served if everyone insists on being the therapist to the neglect of other roles. Especially with the most difficult and disabled patients, specialists with unique skills are needed as members of clinical teams, and the everyone-can-do-everything attitude leads to poor treatment.

Implications for Training and Continuing Education

To further the goals described above, psychiatric residency programs should stress the broad integrative frame of reference we have described, allocating enough time to training in general medicine and neurology so that its graduates are competent to evaluate the interactions between those specialties and psychiatry. Residents should learn the basics of psychodynamic, psychosocial, and psychobiological theories and their scientific underpinnings. The tendency of some current academic programs to limit research and teaching to neurobiology is shortsighted. The psychopharmacologist who avoids learning broader psychiatric skills will be shortchanging his or her patients. Programs should therefore stress training in the three basic, unique characteristics of the profession, emphasizing skills in establishing a therapeutic alliance, the clinical interview, differential diagnosis, and integrating biopsychosocial approaches. Currently, some programs do not.

Since most psychiatrists will spend some professional time in

organized mental health settings, specific training in team participation and team leadership should be part of all residency programs. This leadership experience should go beyond supervising
medical students and junior residents. There should also be adequate exposure to the strengths of other mental health disciplines
so that psychiatrists can be in a position to state not only what
patients need, but also who can best carry out the required tasks.

Continuing medical education opportunities for psychiatrists
should evolve a basic track emphasizing primary skills. This track
would include relevant advances in general medicine, ways to
improve the patient-physician relationship (therapeutic alliance),
new diagnostic techniques, and new advances in the sciences that
would enhance the synthesis of treatment approaches. Current
examples of synthesis are the use of combined psychosocial and
psychopharmacological approaches with schizophrenia, the use of
psychodynamic concepts in enhancing lithium compliance with
bipolar patients, and combining the use of biological markers with
psychodynamics in diagnosis and treatment.

The training of new psychiatrists and the continuing education
of practicing psychiatrists should further strengthen our identity as
physicians willing to take responsibility for treating patients with
mental illnesses. Teaching the unique characteristics of psychiatry
should increase our diagnostic acumen and our familiarity with
the wide range of knowledge in biological, social, and psychological sciences.

By keeping the "T" model in mind, psychiatrists will have a
guideline regarding areas of knowledge that are important to their
practice and will be in a better position to insure that the quality of
their practice meets necessary standards.

To the extent that we can influence general medical training, we
should stress the importance of teaching primary care physicians
the effective use of the physician-patient relationship, the early
recognition of mental illness, the place of psychiatric consultation
in their diagnosis and management of the mentally ill, and the
criteria for referral of their patients to psychiatrists.

Implications for Research

The future of psychiatry depends upon the continued growth of new information resulting from expanded basic and clinical research in biological, dynamic, and social areas of psychiatry. As psychiatry is perceived more as a medical specialty dealing with sick people whose illnesses cost our country billions of dollars annually, funding for such research will become easier. At this time, research in neurobiology is particularly promising, but we must be careful not to ignore recent advances in psychodynamic theory or other aspects of mental functioning in our current enthusiasm for findings in the biological arena. It may be that psychiatry's major contribution will be the integration of the field.

Our recommendations regarding new roles should also be examined with rigorous scientific scrutiny. We will need studies to explore how changes in the role of psychiatrists alter the accessibility and quality of treatment for the mentally ill. While it seems reasonable that psychiatric patients will be better served when primary psychiatrists prescribe treatments, that hypothesis must be tested. Especially important to test are our notions that psychiatrists can contribute to better treatment of those patients we described as living on the streets, seen in primary-care settings, seen by other disciplines, or whose treatment is curtailed by insurance companies or other third-party payors. Research on both the effectiveness and efficiency of all psychiatric treatments (see Chapter 6) is particularly welcome. As new forms of service delivery are considered (such as preferred provider organizations), we should study the most useful roles for psychiatrists, particularly with respect to their primary psychiatric functions.

Implications for Public Policy

We will not stand on a firm foundation in presenting psychiatric roles to the public until we ourselves are clear about how to describe our own identity, direction, and standards. As psychiatry moves in the directions we have suggested, adopting the concepts of primary psychiatrists and psychiatric subspecialists, the public will have greater assurance as to the boundaries of psychiatric illness, in contrast to primarily educational, psychological, and social problems. As standards evolve that hold primary psychiatrists accountable for determining efficiency as well as effectiveness of our treatments, the public will be reassured that their health dollar is being well spent. As psychiatrists demonstrate the effectiveness of a sophisticated physician-patient relationship in providing humane treatment of chronic mental illness, the public will more likely understand the importance of conceptualizing the seriously, chronically mentally ill as patients who need psychiatric physicians, rather than as "clients" needing only "providers." *As the psychiatric profession emphasizes its unique characteristics and its identity with medicine, the public will be in a better position to understand the differences between psychiatry and the other disciplines involved in mental health care.*

Summary and Conclusions

This Report aims to sharpen the focus of psychiatry's contemporary and future identity as a vital medical specialty. Just as mental illness is no myth, so the uniquely comprehensive medical expertise of psychiatric physicians in diagnosing and treating mental illness is no myth.

It is crucial that psychiatrists are physicians: They have passed through the full rigors of medical training. Their clinical experience in this training prepares them to accept the full weight of responsibility for the care of patients, including those who may be seriously, even mortally ill. Their orientation as physicians gives them an appreciation of the enormously complex interactions among biology, personal experience, and social behavior in health and disease. It also attunes them to normal and abnormal human development. No nonphysician has this combination of preparation and skills in medical, psychological, and social sciences and in the understanding and management of doctor-patient relationships.

It is crucial that psychiatrists are specialized physicians: As a result of specialty training, psychiatric physicians bring to both the diagnosis and treatment of the mentally ill a breadth of vision and a depth of relevant detailed knowledge, duplicated neither by other physician-colleagues nor members of other professional groups such as clinical psychologists, social workers, or psychiatric/mental health nurses. There is no shortcut to this kind of competence. Blurring distinctions between professional groups involved in the care of the mentally ill does not serve patients' best interests. Clear role differentiation makes for quality of care.

What psychiatrists bring to the diagnosis and treatment of the mentally ill is uniquely useful, not readily replaced, and also currently underutilized, underappreciated and underfunded.

1. Most patients diagnosed as having a mental illness are initially seen in the primary care sector. More access to specialized care from psychiatrists is required to improve the care of these patients. The establishment of appropriate patterns of medical cooperation and referral with colleagues in primary care should be a major interest of psychiatry. Augmented access to specialized psychiatric care can be provided in a cost-effective manner. Appropriate provision of psychiatric care can, in many settings, produce important savings in the cost of other medical services.

2. A very large number of the sickest mentally ill patients are destitute and totally excluded from appropriate psychiatric care as a consequence of the unbalanced pursuit of deinstitutionalization as a social goal. These patients urgently need the benefits of stable long-term physician-patient relationships with treating psychiatrists. An adequate response to this crisis will require change in the social arrangements governing the care for the incapacitated chronically mentally ill.

3. Economic barriers to an appropriate level of psychiatric care are an important factor in producing suboptimal care for large sectors of the patient population. Funding for the treatment of mental illness needs to be on a par with funding for all other medical illness. Substance abuse, affective disorders, and schizophrenia, for example, have enormous attached morbidity and social costs. It is shortsighted, wasteful, and dangerous to discriminate against the care of patients with these illnesses.

The core of contemporary psychiatric competence is the ability to perform comprehensive diagnosis and treatment planning based on a near state-of-the-art awareness of diagnostic and therapeutic alternatives.

These "primary psychiatric" functions are essential services that, ideally, should be available to every patient in whom mental illness is suspected. Before a patient is treated with a specific regimen or technique, he or she should receive the benefit of such a comprehensive diagnostic and treatment planning evaluation.

New knowledge about mental illnesses and their treatment is being accumulated at a fast pace. Epidemiology, diagnosis, and treatment are much more specific and accountable than they have been in the past. As scientific knowledge about mental illness continues to increase and therapeutic strategies become more refined and specific, increasing subspecialization within psychiatry is bound to occur. Subspecialization should optimally be sanctioned along lines related to patient populations and valid diagnostic groupings, not according to specific therapeutic techniques and theoretical orientations. That is to say, a subspecialty focused on mental disorders among children or on affective illness would be preferable to one based on, say, psychopharmacology, behavior therapy, or psychoanalysis. Psychiatrists who do not feel that they retain this "primary" diagnostic and treatment planning capacity because of their concentration on a special technique or area of expertise should ensure that their patients are seen by a colleague for an initial diagnostic and treatment planning evaluation. There is no reason that a subspecialist cannot also maintain the broader diagnostic and treatment planning skills of a "primary psychiatrist."

Psychiatry bears a special responsibility for maintaining an effective leadership position in the care of the mentally ill. Erosion of such a powerful leadership position does not serve the real interests of today's many patients with disabling mental illnesses.

With many issues regarding mental health care now being actively addressed in political chambers and in executive suites, psychiatrists must become strong and vocal advocates for the mentally ill; actively educate the public and the media about mental illness, its recognition, and treatment; and be willing to take the initiative in designing new systems of mental health care that both protect the quality of treatment of mental patients and at the same time recognize the national mandate to control costs. We have affected public policy in the past and can do so again.

We have a sense of excitement about what psychiatry knows and has to offer patients today and what it will know and have to offer them in the near future. The challenge for psychiatrists is to bring together the best of social, psychological, and biological practices within research, administrative, and especially clinical frameworks of medical practice. There is no other discipline better trained to assume this challenge.

Reference

American Psychiatric Association. *Diagnostic and Statistical Manual of Mental Disorders* (3rd ed.). Washington, DC: Author, 1980.

APPENDICES

In developing this Report concerning new roles for psychiatrists, the committee invited representatives from clinical psychology, clinical social work, and psychiatric/mental health nursing to work with us in exploring interactions among our professions. These discussions, occurring over several years of joint work, served to teach us a great deal about our useful interactions. Sometimes we modified each other's opinion, and those modifications are reflected in the Report. In many areas, however, our disagreements were emphasized and sharpened.

The main body of this report was written by our GAP committee, all psychiatrists. As agreed, we have appended here the chapters written by our three consultants, about their own views of their respective fields. You will see that they disagree with our conclusions in various ways, especially in their insistence on autonomy and their disagreement with our views about the place of psychiatry in diagnosing illness and planning appropriate treatment.

Despite these remaining areas of disagreement, we found our work together—thinking, arguing, and laughing—always stimulating. We are grateful for their good-humored participation in the creation of this Report.

APPENDIX A

CLINICAL PSYCHOLOGY: PROFESSION AND SCIENCE

by George Stricker, Ph.D.

Clinical psychology is only one of the specialty areas of psychology that is involved in the provision of health care services, and health care providers are only one subgroup of psychologists, representing slightly less than half of the people trained in psychology. Counseling psychologists and school psychologists, among others, also provide health services, and a wide variety of other psychologists who do not provide direct services contribute to the basic science of psychology. For the purposes of this report, however, the words "psychologist," "clinical psychologist," and "health care psychologist" will be used interchangeably, but this should not be taken to imply that they are synonymous.

Basic Tenets

Clinical psychology is an autonomous health care profession that remains rooted in the academic discipline of psychology so that it is both a profession and a science. The basic tenets of the profession are threefold. The first tenet is that psychology is an autonomous profession. While every attempt will be made to relate to other professions in a collegial manner, ultimate responsibility for

George Stricker, Ph.D., is Professor and Dean, Adelphi University, Garden City, NY.

psychological services rests with the individual provider. The second tenet is that psychology is a health care profession. This tenet focuses on the concern of psychology on being responsive to the entire range of health problems that the patient may present, within the boundaries set by the professional competence of the provider. Traditionally, these problems have been primarily in the areas of mental health, but psychologists are increasingly becoming involved with a wide variety of other health conditions, recognizing that these have significant emotional components. There is, of course, no intention to provide medical intervention, but there is a recognition that physical intervention alone is insufficient to remedy many of the major health problems that beset our populace. The third tenet is that psychology is a science. This has two important implications. The first involves the training of psychologists. This training includes a thorough grounding in many areas of the behavioral sciences that bear on the development or amelioration of health problems. In addition, psychology's scientific roots provide a concern with the outcome of the services as well as the process, and this leads to a recognition of the need for accountability to the public and to the profession.

Functional Definition

The *Standards for Providers of Psychological Services* (American Psychological Association [APA], 1977) includes an explicit definition of the range of psychological services as follows:

1. Evaluation, diagnosis, and assessment of the functioning of individuals and groups in a variety of settings and activities.
2. Interventions to facilitate the functioning of individuals and groups. Such interventions may include psychological counseling, psychotherapy, and process consultation.
3. Consultation relating to 1 and 2 above.
4. Program development services in the areas of 1, 2, and 3 above.
5. Supervision of psychological services.

Training

Training in psychology culminates in the doctoral degree. The necessity of the doctoral degree for the practice of psychology has been asserted numerous times by the profession and has been upheld, after an investigation, by the Civil Service Commission (1978). This latter group produced a study that found that the doctoral degree was an appropriate credential for civil service psychologist positions at the independent level. Psychologists also have the opportunity to engage in postdoctoral clinical training. Both Adelphi University and the New York University offer post-doctoral training programs, and a number of institutions independent of a university setting also admit psychologists to advanced training programs.

Historically, training in psychology has been conducted within a scientist-practitioner model, which was initially stated at the Boulder conference (Raimy, 1950) and has since been reaffirmed at every major national conference that was concerned with graduate education in psychology (Cutts, 1955; Hoch, Ross, & Winder, 1966; Korman, 1973; Roe, Gustad, Moore, Ross, & Skodak, 1959; Thompson & Super, 1964). Most recently, however, at the Vail conference (Korman, 1973) endorsement was also given to an alternative model for training. The practitioner model relies on a basic service orientation in a context of scientific scholarship, but without the same rigorous attention to scientific training. Although the practitioner model focuses on the development of applied skills, it does so with a clear commitment to the science of psychology as the source of the substantive basis of the education and training programs. The scientist-practitioner programs all result in the award of the Ph.D. degree, while practitioner programs may award either the Ph.D. or the Psy.D. degree.

The most comprehensive account of the nature of training in clinical psychology can be garnered by studying the *Criteria for Accreditation of Doctoral Training Programs and Internships in Professional Psychology* (APA, 1979). The curriculum of a program requires a minimum of three full-time academic years of resident graduate study. Within this program, the student must be instructed in "scientific and professional ethics and standards, research design and methodology, statistics, psychological measurement, and history and systems of psychology" (p. 6). In addition, the student must demonstrate competence in each of the following substantive content areas:

1. Biological bases of behavior (e.g., physiological psychology, comparative psychology, neuropsychology, sensation, psychopharmacology);
2. Cognitive-affective bases of behavior (e.g., learning, memory, perception, cognition, thinking, motivation, emotion);
3. Social bases of behavior (e.g., social psychology; cultural, ethnic and group processes; sex roles; organizational and systems theory);
4. Individual behavior (e.g., personality theory, human development, individual differences, abnormal psychology). (p. 6)

In addition to these academic requirements, the students are also required to have training in particular skills that are related to their areas of specialization, and these skills must be broad based, rather than restricted to a single method or orientation. The students are also instructed in the values of professional and scientific responsibility and integrity. The course of study usually culminates in the production of a major research product, such as a doctoral dissertation, which will be relevant to the student's training and interest.

Every clinical psychology training program requires that the student complete a full year internship. This internship is also subject to accreditation by the American Psychological Association. The internship provides the trainee with the opportunity to take substantial responsibility for carrying out major professional functions, while also assuring appropriate supervision and role modeling. It serves as a means of preparing the student for functioning as an independent professional.

Sites for Practice

Clinical psychologists can be found at any type of facility that offers health services to the public. They provide outpatient services in clinics and CMHCs as well as in private individual and group practice. They provide inpatient services at federal facilities, such as the Veterans Administration hospitals, state and county hospitals, and also private mental hospitals. They can be found providing liaison services in general hospitals, as well as working on psychiatric wings of general hospitals. Psychologists also work in residential treatment centers and in rehabilitation centers.

Aside from providing clinical services, psychologists are also involved in the administration of mental health programs. They can serve as directors of most of the facilities in which they provide services. Psychologists are involved in the administration of CMHCs, psychiatric hospitals, outpatient clinics, mental retardation programs, and rehabilitation programs. They work in important positions in many federal agencies and also as commissioners and directors of many state agencies and departments.

In keeping with the role of psychology as a science, many psychologists are also involved in education, training, and research settings. A large number of psychologists are on the faculty of universities and professional schools, where they contribute to the training of graduate students in psychology. In addition, psychologists are included in research, clinical, or academic capacities on the faculty of professional schools in other disciplines such as medicine, dentistry, nursing, and social work. A number of psychologists are employed by private or governmental agencies in primarily research positions, where their contribution is to our knowledge of health care services and health delivery systems.

Licensure and Certification

Psychologists are subject to licensure and certification in all 50 states and in the District of Columbia. Typically, these are certification laws that protect the title "psychologist" but do not restrict the practice of psychology. While laws differ from state to state, most laws require a doctoral degree, two years of supervised experience, and an examination procedure for licensure. The examination recognizes that the practice of psychology is based upon the science of psychology and includes basic science as well as practice questions.

Psychology is similar to other professions in that its license is generic. The state does not recognize specialty practice, but it remains the responsibility of the profession to determine who is competent to offer health services. The *Standards for Providers of Psychological Services* clearly indicates that psychologists should limit their practice to their specific areas of expertise. In the event that a psychologist trained in one area wishes to practice in another, a separate standard is responsive to this desire for lateral mobility. It states, "Psychologists who wish to change their service specialty or to add an additional area of applied specialization must meet the same requirements with respect to subject matter and professional skills that apply to doctoral training in the new specialty" (APA, 1977, p. 3). In response to this requirement, a number of universities have developed respecialization programs in order to help the psychologist who wishes to move from one specialty area into another.

One method by which the public may be made aware of which psychologists are trained to provide health services is the *National Register of Health Service Providers in Psychology* (Council for the National Register. . ., 1981). The Register is used in two different ways by the insurance industry: First, many insurance programs list the National Register directly as prima facie evidence of eligibility to provide services; second, since this is a voluntary listing, they may list criteria that are the substantial equivalent of those of the National Register as an alternative means toward receiving authorization to provide services. Basically, these criteria include state licensure, a doctoral degree from a regionally accredited university and two years of supervised experience in health services, at least one of which must have been postdoctoral.

By means of state licensure, internal professional surveillance, and the National Register, a psychologist may be licensed generically and identified to the public as practicing within the specialty area of health service delivery.

Strengths of Specialty

The primary strength of psychology is linked to its development as a science as well as a profession. The ongoing scientific training of psychologists and the integration of science with practice, rather than the separation of science training and clinical training, contribute to the mode of practice eventually adopted by psychologists. The implication of this approach to training can be seen in a number of important ways. Because the training in research and practice is integrated, it is not unusual to find a psychologist who is active in both areas. If there is no separation between basic science and clinical practice, there can be a process by which one area informs the other so that the research will become relevant to clinical concerns and the clinical practice can be based on research findings. Many research activities of psychologists have led directly to clinical contributions. This interrelationship is most apparent with the development of the behavior therapies, although it is not restricted to that approach. It should be noted that research is not only used for the development of new approaches, but also for the evaluation of existing approaches. Psychologists place great empirical demand upon their practice, and their training leads them to look for evidence of efficacy in empirical data rather than anecdotal speculation.

As a profession, psychology is at least as much involved with community practice as it is with private practice. Less than half the health care psychologists are engaged in full-time private practice (Dorken & Webb, 1979a; Gottfredson & Dyer, 1978). There is a substantial commitment by psychologists to provide services in community settings where they can reach the underserved and the disadvantaged. Psychologists also function effectively in private practice, but this does not constitute their highest priority.

Because psychology is not primarily oriented toward individual private practice, the contributions of its practitioners have been able to express more concern for community issues and to reflect more of a public health orientation. Active models of intervention have been adopted, as a contract to the passive orientation of the private practitioner. Preventive programs have been encouraged, with the hope that a major impact could be made on large populations rather than on single, needy individuals. A systems conceptualization of pathology has been possible, with a resultant recommendation for intervention at points in the system other than the single suffering patient.

Psychology has voiced some resentment about being defined in terms of what it is not rather than what it is. For example, the legislation creating Professional Standards Review Organizations groups psychologists with a large number of other professions, referring to them all as nonphysician health care providers or health care providers other than physicians (Public Law 92-603, 1972). Curiously, however, this lack of identity with medicine is the source of a great strength for psychology. Training does not occur within a disease model, and this removes a number of constraints on conceptualization of health care and health delivery. This is not to say that psychologists do not contribute to developments within the traditional model. Growing advances in clinical neuropsychology (Boll, 1978) underline the contribution of psychologists in a classic area of mental health related dysfunction, and psychologists have been increasingly active in providing general health care services outside of the mental health domain (Wright, 1976). Some of the unique contributions of psychology, however, have occurred in a manner that demonstrates its freedom from the disease model.

Psychology, for example, is not committed to a taxonomic formulation of dysfunction. Medicine traditionally has focused on systems of classification, which have been an appropriate and, at times, crucial step in providing proper treatment for patients. The primary assumption underlying a diagnostic approach is that diagnosis dictates treatment, so that without a clear diagnostic formulation an adequate therapeutic regimen could not be assigned. The validity of this assumption in the mental health arena is subject to serious question. For example, if one examines the review criteria adopted by professional standards review organizations (American Medical Association [AMA], 1975), one is immediately struck by the extraordinary amount of redundancy. While criteria are established in terms of diagnosis, these criteria are virtually identical from diagnosis to diagnosis, with the exception of some pharmacological interventions.

Blum (1978) has recently found that diagnoses have changed over the past two decades, showing a sharp reduction in hospitalized neuroses and a sharp increase in hospitalization for affective disorders and schizophrenia. A careful analysis suggests that one probable explanation for this shift is that diagnosis follows, rather than precedes, treatment. Thus, when the treatment of choice was psychoanalytic psychotherapy, the diagnosis of choice was neurosis. As pharmacological interventions have been developed, the same patient might receive a diagnosis of affective disorder or schizophrenia, thereby justifying the treatment that was being offered. A move toward a more problem-oriented basis of case formation would not lose any information and would offer the advantage of a new perspective on the patient.

Finally, freedom from a disease model also allows freedom from a reliance on hospitalization as the necessary alternative to outpatient care. Psychologists have been active in the development of alternative care facilities as meaningful options for a patient in need of treatment (Stein & Test, 1978). The use of day-care programs, halfway houses, apartment living programs, and other transitional facilities represent means of providing treatment that are at least equally effective and far less costly than traditional hospital care.

Weakness of Specialty

Psychology has a number of weaknesses that can be located within the profession itself. Since licensure is generic, it allows for practice outside of the psychologist's area of specialty training. Individuals trained, for instance, in experimental psychology, may enter into the practice of clinical psychology, particularly as economic conditions restrict opportunities outside the service delivery areas. Such practice is considered unethical; it violates many statutory regulations, but nevertheless it does occur.

Although psychology prides itself on being a science profession, with its values and practices derived from that identity, many individual practitioners in psychology, as in other mental health professions, neglect the scientific basis of practice in favor of a more artistic approach. Not only do most practitioners fail to conduct and publish research, some are not even active consumers of research.

Because psychology is a science profession, training can be uneven. Some training programs place emphasis on science, with less rigorous and intensive practice experience, while others are much more practice oriented. A Ph.D. in psychology indicates a basic core of common training but does not guarantee the extent of the specialty training beyond the core.

In the process of training, psychologists are exposed to a wide variety of practicum experiences. Many of these are in outpatient settings, and those in hospital settings often suffer from restrictions in scope of practice. As a result, critical responsibility for life and death decisions are not usually part of the training experience, and it would add to the function of the professional to have had this background.

The primary weaknesses of psychology, however, result from artificial external barriers that impede its ability to function as an independent and self-regulating profession. The two major areas where these barriers exist are in the hospital and with respect to third-party payment (O'Keefe & McCullough, 1979). The hospital barriers are created by the Joint Commission for the Accreditation of Hospitals (JCAH), while the health insurance barriers are created in large part by the actions of Blue Cross and Blue Shield. While neither JCAH nor the Blues represent any other profession directly, both seem to be dominated by medical interests, and the clashes have led to a number of current actions which are still being actively considered in the courts.

While JCAH is not a regulatory agency, it has been given status in so many different pieces of legislation that it functions as a quasi-legal entity. JCAH insists that physicians control all activities within hospital settings or JCAH will threaten to withhold accreditations from the hospital. Thus, if the standards were followed exactly, psychologists would not be able to admit or discharge patients, provide independent services, write orders, enter comments on patient charts, or vote on policy-making committees. While psychologists do perform some of these functions in a small number of hospitals (Dorken & Webb, 1979b), they do so in violation of JCAH regulations. Those regulations do assign a service function to psychologists, but they require the direct supervision of a physician.

The situation with regard to third-party payment is often dependent upon state legislation and the private action of insurance companies. In over half the states, with almost three-quarters of the population, direct recognition statutes assure that psychologists can function as independent providers. Unfortunately, in the states without direct recognition statutes, and in some federal programs such as Medicare and Medicaid, recognition for psychologists may require physician supervision.

It is clear that a requirement for physician supervision of psychologists, whether it be in the hospital or in the private sector, is a weakness of the profession and is inimical to the interests of psychologists. More important, however, this required supervision is also inimical to the interest of consumers, who find that they must contract for time-consuming, costly, and unnecessary services. It should be clear that we are not referring to the often necessary consultation that a psychologist might seek with a medical colleague in order to best serve the needs of the patient. Rather, we are referring to required supervision by a member of one profession over services offered by a member of another profession, even though the person for whom supervision is required is fully qualified, trained, and licensed to practice independently. A more full recognition of psychology's role as an autonomous profession would be helpful to psychologists, but it would be far more important in its contribution to an efficient and well-functioning health care system.

There is one additional area in which psychologists may not function, by virtue of both legal restriction and absence of training. This is the area involving the prescription of medication. While this is a weakness of the profession, in a curious way it also contributes to a strength, because it encourages psychologists to look beyond pharmacology for solutions to some problems of living. Psychologists will recognize the need and seek consultation in the event that medication is necessary but they are hampered by their inability to act directly. Their first response to a problem, however, will not be to medicate it, and in some instances this will redound to the advantage of the patient. Nevertheless, psychologists would be in a better position to provide a full range of health care options if their training would include psychopharmacology and the statutes would allow them to practice in this area.

Work Patterns

The great majority of psychologists do not restrict themselves to practice in a single setting. The number of psychologists who list either individual or group private practice as their primary work setting varies between 20% and 50%, with the estimate seeming to increase with each passing year. Approximately 10% of health psychologists list universities as their primary work settings, and an additional 10% list CMHCs as their primary setting. Psychologists work over 40 hours a week and spend approximately half their time in the delivery of health services. An additional third of their time is involved in education, management, and administration, with the balance devoted to research and other professional activities. It has been estimated that over one million patients are seen by psychologists in private practice each year, and at least that many are seen by psychologists in organized health care settings. Clearly, psychologists make a major contribution to the provision of health care services to people in need of treatment.

Private Practice

It is quite difficult to estimate the number of psychologists who are currently active in private practice. It is possible to identify four separate groups of psychologists but quite difficult to determine how many are in each group. There are some psychologists who are in full-time private practice, a large number of others who are in part-time private practice, a third group who offer health care services on a salaried basis in an institutional setting, but not in private practice, and a fourth group qualified to offer health services, but not presently doing so. Psychologists can move back and forth among these groups so that, at any one point, it is difficult to determine precise figures. This situation, however, makes very clear the elasticity of the supply of psychologists in private practice. The current amount of service being offered represents a minimum, since so many other psychologists are qualified to offer services and could expand the involvement in private practice, if the need should arise. This elasticity represents a great strength of the profession, since psychology is capable of increasing the services it offers to the public by a very substantial amount without any increase in training facilities or reduction in quality of service.

The qualifications of psychologists to offer independent services in private practice have been widely recognized. The federal government has recognized psychologists in its Federal Employees Health Benefits Program, its Civilian Health and Medical Program for the Uniform Services, its Workmen's Compensation Act, and its Vocational Rehabilitation Act. The state governments have recognized psychologists as autonomous providers in a number of Direct Recognition statutes, in the provisions of a number of Mandatory Minimal Mental Health Coverage acts, in a large number of Medicaid plans, and in some Workmen's Compensation acts. A number of private employers have also provided for direct recognition of psychologists in their industry health plans. For example, companies such as Delta Airlines and groups such as the United Rubber Workers have provided for the independent reimbursement of psychologists.

Perhaps the most concise way of summarizing the potential role of psychologists in private practice is to quote from a classic work by an eminent psychiatrist. Dr. Lewis Wolberg, in Part I of *The Technique of Therapy* (1967), cited a conclusion that "taking into consideration the total graduate education, specialty training, and supervision, it would seem doubtful that psychologists are exceeded by any other mental health profession in the extensiveness of preparation for the private practice of psychotherapy" (p. 324).

Hospital Practice

The role of psychologists in an inpatient setting is far more limited than their ability to offer services would suggest (Dorken & Webb, 1979b). A large majority of psychologists do not provide any direct service to hospital inpatients. This probably can be traced to the very small proportion of psychologists who have been granted clinical privileges or, even less likely, granted formal membership on hospital staffs. This suggests a lack of acceptance of psychologists in the hospital setting, which can be traced directly to the regulations of the Joint Commission on Accreditation of Hospitals. This policy is not in keeping with the best interests of patients, who can avail themselves of psychological services on an outpatient, but not an inpatient, basis. This lack of acceptance of the clinical contributions of psychologists is particularly curious since, in 1976, 2,336 psychologists served on 115 medical school faculties in this country (Matarazzo, Lubin, & Nathan, 1978).

Outpatient Settings

Psychologists have been quite active in organized outpatient settings, both in service provision and in administrative roles. In CMHCs, between 1972 and 1976, psychologists had a higher percentage increase in positions than any other health care discipline and also assumed the directorship in a large number of these settings. In HMOs the pattern of psychologists' involvement is highly variable. While some exclude psychologists, others are staffed almost in total by psychologists. It is interesting to note the variety of roles that psychologists have adopted in the HMO setting (Sank & Shapiro, 1979). Other than traditional clinical service roles, psychologists have been active in a variety of administrative, liaison, educational, and research activities, which allow for the provision of a full range of health services. The success that psychologists have had in providing this spectrum of services in an HMO suggests the vast untapped resources that they represent for the hospital setting. In any case, settings that have accepted psychologists have found them to be valuable and actively contributing members of the service staff.

Relationship with Other Core Disciplines

Psychologists have attempted to preserve cordial, cooperative, and collegial relations with members of other professions, while at the same time preserving their own professional autonomy. There is a portion of the Ethics Code (APA, 1981) that is specifically relevant to professional relationships, and this reads, "Psychologists act with due regard for the needs, special competencies and obligations of their colleagues in psychology and other professions" (p. 3). Subprinciples include statements that "Psychologists understand the areas of competence of related professions. They make full use of all the professional, technical, and administrative resources that serve the best interests of consumers. . . . Psychologists know and take into account the traditions and practices of other professional groups with whom they work and cooperate fully with such groups" (p. 3). In addition, the *Criteria for Accreditation of Doctoral Training Programs* includes a specific requirement that students must be given access to appropriate instruction in fields such as the biological and social sciences (APA, 1979).

It is of note that psychologists maintain a reasonable pattern of exchanging referrals with members of other professions (Dorken & Webb, 1979a). In a recent survey 28% of psychologists indicated that their primary source of referral was nonpsychiatric physicians, and an additional 17% had psychiatrists as their primary referral source. When psychologists refer patients, 22% indicated that they often referred to nonpsychiatric physicians, and 16% often refer to psychiatrists. In practice, then, there seems to be a readiness for psychologists to recognize the special competency of other professionals, and, in turn, to be recognized by them.

Psychology's position is defined by a sense of autonomy and respect for the autonomy of others. It would be naive to overlook the current conflict that is occurring on a number of legislative and legal fronts between psychology and medicine (O'Keefe & McCullough, 1979). These conflicts are often the result of one profession's attempt to define the scope of responsibilities of the other. Too often, the nature of the conflict confuses guild interests with public interests, and it is unlikely that any uninvolved mediator will act in a manner that will further either profession's self-interest. There may be legitimate differences in perception as to where the best interest of the patient lies, but that should be the focus of the resolution of professional disputes. Psychology wishes to act in the public interest and is quite willing to act cooperatively with other disciplines, but it will insist on preserving its own autonomy, as long as that is consistent with the public welfare.

References

American Medical Association. *Model Screening Criteria to Assist Professional Standards Review Organizations.* Chicago: Author, 1975.

American Psychological Association. *Criteria for Accreditation of Doctoral Training Programs and Internships in Professional Psychology.* Washington, DC: Author, 1979.

American Psychological Association. *Ethical Standards of Psychologists* (rev. ed.). Washington, DC: Author, 1981.

American Psychological Association. *Standards for Providers of Psychological Services.* Washington, DC: Author, 1977.

Blum, J.D. On changes in psychiatric diagnosis over time. *American Psychologist,* 33:1017–1031, 1978.

Boll, T.J. Diagnosing brain impairment. In B.B. Wolman (Ed.), *Clinical Diagnosis of Mental Disorders.* New York: Plenum, 1978.

Civil Service Commission. *Job Relatedness Study of the Doctoral Degree Requirement for Clinical Psychologist Positions.* Washington, DC: Author, 1978.

Council for the National Register of Health Service Providers in Psychology. *National Register of Health Service Providers in Psychology.* Washington, DC: Author, 1981.

Cutts, N. (Ed.). *School Psychologists at Midcentury: A Report on the Thayer Conference on the Functions, Qualifications, and Training of School Psychologists.* Washington, DC: American Psychological Association, 1955.

Dorken, H., & Webb, J. Licensed psychologists in health care: A survey of their practices. In C. Kiesler, N. Cummings, & G. VandenBos (Eds.), *Psychology and National Health Insurance: A Sourcebook.* Washington, DC: American Psychological Association, 1979a.

Dorken, H., & Webb, J. The hospital practice of psychology: An interstate comparison. *Professional Psychology,* 10:619–630, 1979b.

Gottfredson, G.D., & Dyer, S.E. Health service providers in psychology. *American Psychologist,* 33:314–338, 1978.

Hoch, E.L., Ross, A.O., & Winder, C.L. (Eds.). *Professional Preparation of Clinical Psychologists.* Washington DC: American Psychological Association, 1966.

Korman, M. (Ed.). *Levels and Patterns of Professional Training in Psychology.* Washington, DC: American Psychological Association, 1973.

Matarazzo, J., Lubin, B., & Nathan, R. Psychologist's membership in the medical staff of university teaching hospitals. *American Psychologist,* 33:23–29, 1978.

O'Keefe, A.M., & McCullough, S.J. Physician domination in the health care industry: The pursuit of antitrust redress. *Professional Psychology,* 10:605–618, 1979.

Public Law 92-603. Ninety second Congress of the United States of America, M.R.1. Washington, DC: US Government Printing Office, October 30, 1972.

Raimy, V.C. (Ed.), *Training in Clinical Psychology.* New York: Prentice-Hall, 1950.

Roe, A., Gustad, J.W., Moore, B.V., Ross, S., & Skodak, M. (Eds.). *Graduate Education in Psychology.* Washington, DC: American Psychological Association, 1959.

Sank, L.I., & Shapiro, J.R. Case examples of the broadened role of psychology in health maintenance organizations. *Professional Psychology,* 10:402–408, 1979.

Stein, L.I., & Test, M.A. (Eds.). *Alternatives to Mental Hospital Treatment.* New York: Plenum, 1978.

Thompson, A.S., & Super, D.E. (Eds.). *The Professional Preparation of Counseling Psychologists.* New York: Columbia University Teachers College, Bureau of Publications, 1964.

Wolberg, L.R. *The Technique of Psychotherapy* (Part I). New York: Grune & Stratton, 1967.

Wright, L. Psychology as a health profession. *Clinical Psychologist,* 29:16–19, 1976.

APPENDIX B

CLINICAL SOCIAL WORK: AN ECOLOGICAL/SYSTEMS PERSPECTIVE

by Florence Segal, A.C.S.W.

Definition of Specialty

Clinical social work is well rooted in the multifaceted profession of social work. Traditionally, social work practitioners have dealt with problems in the realm of interaction between people and their environments, practicing in varied fields, with varied populations, and utilizing different theories of practice while providing direct services to people, as well as planning, organizing, and administering services.

The primary theoretical orientation of clinical social work is an ecological or social systems orientation, incorporating understanding of an individual as a biopsychosocial system and interacting with a network of individuals and social systems (Northern, 1982). Many clinical social workers practice within a synthesized theoretical orientation of system theory, role theory, psychoanalytic theory, and ego psychology. The term "clinical social worker" is of fairly recent origin, apparently formally used first in the California State Licensing Law of 1968. It is now interesting to note the number of advertisements in both professional journals and newspapers adver-

Florence Segal, A.C.S.W., is Director of Continuing Education, School of Social Work, Virginia Commonwealth University, Richmond, VA.

tising for clinical social workers. Frequently, the term seems to be used as a substitute for "psychiatric social worker."

Before 1968 psychiatric social work was clearly defined as a specific field of practice within the professional orbit of social work. The specificity grew out of the "application of social work skills in hospital or clinic settings where the psychiatric specialty of medicine is practiced," (Berkman, p. 5) or "social work practice in direct and responsible working relationships with psychiatry"; "it occurs in hospitals, clinics or other psychiatric auspices which serve people with mental or emotional disorders" *Education for Psychiatric Social Work,* 1950). Now the term "clinical social worker" serves as a unifying concept for many of those who used to be called psychiatric social workers, those practitioners in private practice, and the thousands of caseworkers in all settings who have concern for and expertise in helping troubled persons with psychosocial problems. It is frequently used to characterize those social workers who practice psychodynamically oriented casework and group therapy. It will be used in this chapter to describe those social workers who are "assisting individuals, families, and groups in dealing with problems of social functioning whether these are caused by internal or external factors. Such problems may be manifested in intrapsychic or interpersonal functioning or they may be reflected in the person's transactions with the environment" (Chestang, 1979). "The objectives of the clinical social worker are both preventive and remedial, and the methods used are varied, including any combination of clinical psychotherapy, group psychotherapy, family therapy, concrete services and interventions on behalf of clients with social systems and the environment" (Pinkus, 1975).

Basic Tenets

The biopsychosocial view of man and society is a basic tenet of clinical social work and supports the idea that the individual must be understood in relation to his environment. Historically, this view was espoused as far back as in the writings of Mary Richmond (1917) and Jane Addams (1918), early pioneers in the social work profession. This tenet mandates that the clinical social worker be concerned "both with the coping qualities of the individual and the impinging dyadic group, organizational, and physical environments (Younghusband, 1964). The view of the individual in a social context is consonant with the practice of clinical social work, which, like all professions is recognized by a constellation of 1) values; 2) purpose; 3) sanctions; 4) knowledge; and 5) method.

Values

The values repeatedly delineated by the profession of social work in the United States are viewed as a melding of certain Judeo-Christian beliefs and concepts enunciated in our constitution. They are paraphrased as follows: the worth and dignity of the individual; society's responsibility to meet the needs of its members; the interdependence of man and society; the right of the individual to pursue his own destiny as long as it does not interfere with the rights of others; the right to privacy (Northern, 1982). The ultimate value of social work is that human beings should have opportunities to realize their potentialities for living in ways that are both personally satisfying and socially desirable. Implicit in this basic value is simultaneous concern for *individual* and *collective* welfare. The value base of social work from a broad psychosocial perspective is "humanistic, scientific, and democratic. It is *humanistic* in its commitment to the welfare of the client, its concern with client participation and decision making in the process, its regard for the client as a whole person, and its commitment to the protection of his rights. It is *scientific* in that it prefers objectivity and factual evidence over personal biases. It emphasizes that the practitioner's judgments and actions are derived from a reasoning process based on scientific knowledge to the extent that it is available" (Woods, 1981).

Values have been discussed by many authors. Those stated

reflect, for the most part, views expressed by Gordon Hamilton (1951), Nathan Cohen (1958), and Helen Harris Perlman (1976).*

Most of the following sections on Purpose, Sanction, Knowledge, and Method are quoted from Bartlett (1958).

Purpose

The practice of social work has as its purposes: 1) to assist individuals and groups to identify and resolve or minimize problems arising out of disequilibrium between themselves and their environments; 2) to identify potential areas of disequilibrium between individuals or groups and the environment in order to prevent occurrence of disequilibrium; 3) . . . to seek out, identify, and strengthen the maximum potential in individuals, groups and communities.

Sanction

Social work has developed out of a community recognition of the necessity to provide services to meet basic needs, services which require the intervention of practitioners trained to understand the services, themselves, the individuals, and the means for bringing these elements together. Social work is not practiced in a vacuum or at the choice of its practitioners alone. . . . The authority and power of the practitioner and what he represents to the clients and group members derive from one or a combination of three sources: 1) *governmental agencies* or their subdivisions (authorized by law); 2) *voluntary incorporated agencies,* which have taken responsibility for meeting certain . . . needs or providing certain services necessary for individual and group welfare; 3) the *organized profession,* which . . . can sanction individuals for the practice of social work and set forth the educational and other requirements for practice and the conditions under which that practice may be undertaken, whether or not carried out under organizational auspices.

---

*For elaboration and further discussion of values in social work and the broader society, the reader is referred to the entire special issue of *Social Casework* (1976, M.M. Mangold, Ed.) entitled "Family Life Today: Critical Issues and Lasting Values," and *Social Work Values in an Age of Discontent* (1970, K. Kendall, Ed.).

Knowledge

Social work, like all other professions, derives knowledge from a variety of sources and in application brings forth further knowledge from its own processes. . . . The practice of the social worker is typically guided by knowledge of: 1) human development and behavior characterized by emphasis on the wholeness of the individual and the reciprocal influences of man and his total environment—human, social, economic, and cultural; 2) the psychology of giving and taking help from another person or source . . . ; 3) ways in which people communicate with one another and give outer expression to inner feelings, such as words, gestures, and activities; 4) group process and the effects of groups upon individuals and the reciprocal influence of the individual upon the group; 5) the meaning and effect on the individual, groups, and community of cultural heritage including its religious beliefs, spiritual values, law, and other social institutions; 6) relationships, that is, the interactional processes between individuals, between individual and groups, and between group and group; 7) the community, its internal processes, modes of development and change, its social services and resources; 8) the social services, their structure, organization, and methods; 9) himself, which enables the individual practitioner to be aware of and take responsibility for his own emotions and attitudes as they affect his professional functions. (pp. 6–7)

Concepts from the biological, psychological, and social sciences are selected for their relevance to the effective use of social work in direct service to people for the achievement of goals within the realm of psychosocial functioning. In addition, the use of general systems theory and an ecological systems perspective provides a broad framework to guide the clincial social worker in observations and assessments of a person/group/situation configuration. Quite recently, the editor of *Social Work,* the journal of the National Association of Social Workers wrote that "clinical social work which focuses only on internal processes in individuals, families, and small groups may be useful and appropriate for some people but it is not within the social work domain" (Minahan, 1980, p. 171). This statement is a controversial one, not embraced by all clinical social workers. Some clinical social workers focus *only* on internal processes as appropriate for all psychotherapists, including clinical social workers.

Method

The social work method is the responsible, conscious, disciplined use of self in a relationship with an individual or group. Through this relationship the practitioner facilitates interaction between the individual and his social environment with a continuing awareness of the reciprocal effects of one upon the other. It facilitates change: 1) within the individual in relation to his social environment; 2) of the social environment in its effect upon the individual; 3) of both the individual and the social environment in their interaction.

Social work method includes systematic observation and assessment of the individual or group in a situation and the formulation of an appropriate plan of action. Implicit in this is a continuing evaluation regarding the nature of the relationship between worker and client or group, and its effect on both the participant individual or group and on the worker himself. This evaluation provides the basis for the professional judgment which the worker must constantly make and which determines the direction of his activities. The method is used predominately in interviews, group sessions, and conferences. (p. 7)

Training/Education

In 1967 the National Association of Social Workers (NASW) adopted a code of ethics that defined social work practice as requiring "mastery of a body of knowledge and skill gained through professional education and experience." The educational system has four levels of formal training—associate, baccalaureate, master's level, and doctoral programs—and the emerging programs of continuing education. B.S.W. and M.S.W. programs are subject to accreditation standards administered by the Council on Social

Work Education. In 1977 there were 84 accredited master's degree programs in the United States and 211 accredited undergraduate programs (Council on Social Work Education, 1978).

There is strong agreement among clinical social workers (e.g., Cooper, 1980) that there must be a clear delineation between the role of B.S.W. graduates and M.S.W. graduates. It is agreed that completion of the master's degree in social work is a necessity for clinical practice. Many in the field of social work have written and spoken about this issue and disagree with others who argue that clinical practice should be relegated to the undergraduate level, while master's level work should aim to develop supervisors, consultants, evaluators, and administrators. The undergraduate program can and does introduce students to the field of social work, to theories of human personality, to sociology, and to practice modalities. It teaches technician skills by demonstrating how to offer certain concrete services, but it cannot systematically educate for clinical proficiency.

In particular, Lawrence Kubie clearly distinguishes between learning about clinical processes as a valid abstract discipline, amenable to classroom and textbook study, and becoming a clinician—a very different learning endeavor (Kubie, 1971). Supporting this point of view is a statement in the Register of Clinical Social Workers issued by the National Association of Social Workers. A listing in the Register requires "a master's or doctoral degree in social work from an accredited graduate school of social work, accredited or recognized by the Council on Social Work Education; two years or three thousand hours of postmaster's supervised clinical social work practice under the supervision of a master's degree social worker, or if social work supervision could be shown to be unavailable, supervision by another mental health professional with the added condition of giving evidence of continued participation and identification within the social work profession" (National Association of Social Workers, 1976, p. xi).

Master's level education is typically a four-term or six-quarter program consisting of 60 credit hours that provide classroom instruction and a field practicum. Many schools offer students the opportunity to choose concentrations in method (e.g., casework, group work, community organization, social planning, administration, research) and in field of practice (e.g., child welfare, criminal justice, family services, mental health services, public assistance, school social work). Classroom instruction consists of courses on social welfare policy and services, human behavior, and the social environment and provides the background for the methods component of the classroom curriculum. Field instruction is offered with the cooperation of the practice community, social agencies, mental health clinics, hospitals, etc., provide instructional services. Field instruction is designed to provide the student with the opportunity to integrate, utilize, and apply content learned in the classroom to problems in practice.

In the curriculum policy statement issued by the Council on Social Work Education,* effective July 1, 1983, the importance of the field practicum as an integral part of the curriculum in social work education was reaffirmed. To accomplish the educational purposes of the practicum, graduate programs were mandated to provide each student with a minimum of 900 hours in a field placement.

Postmaster's programs are beginning to develop for social workers, and doctoral education is on the increase, with most doctoral programs focusing on preparation for teaching, research, and/or planning or administration rather than on direct clinical practice. In addition, a few schools of social work are beginning to develop postmaster's certificate training programs through their continuing education departments. This latter development is consonant with the renewed thrust toward direct clinical practice by social workers and in response to the proliferation of social work licensing regulations in the United States.

Licensing

A current issue that serves as an impetus for strengthening the focus on clinical social work is the issue of licensing. In 1915 Justice

---

*Distributed to members by the Council. For further information write to the Council at 111 Eighth Avenue, New York, NY, 10011.

Felix Frankfurter held that social work was a definable profession requiring special training like law and medicine. Fundamental to such a definition is the acceptance of the concept that the social worker is capable of being an independent practitioner, even though he works under institutional auspices. In their study of the future of clinical practice, Grinnell and Kyte (1977) concluded that their findings "appear to provide strong measure of support for recent predictions of the swing in social work toward clinical practice" (p. 137). Of the 1,082 graduate and undergraduate social work students studied, 53.2% (31.9%, 15.9%, and 5.4% respectively) designated casework, psychotherapy, or private practice as their ideal career choice. There is no doubt that the trend observed in 1977 has continued and expanded. Clinical social workers are being licensed by more and more states.

A profession is validated through licensure and through the legislative process. It is granted recognition by governmental action as a recognizable and definable entity that should have its members' practice regulated in the public interest. The legitimate function of licensure is to protect the public from incompetent and unqualified practitioners and to identify the qualified practitioners.

Members of the profession have been and continue to be in conflict about the question of licensing and, until recently, disagreed about the desirability of even being licensed. Currently, the idea of social work licensing seems to have gained general acceptance, but now the question of who will be licensed to do what has stimulated fierce intraprofessional battles—battles that still rage and are far from being resolved.

Professional confusions have been mirrored in the confusion of legislators and their reluctance to support the licensing of a nonrigidly defined profession. "Pragmatically, for the profession to survive, licensing is essential as it is the foundation on which many other matters rest." These include third-party vendor payments, inclusion in National Health Insurance and Public Law 92-603, and efforts by the federal government to establish quality control on behalf of consumers of Medicare, Medicaid, and Maternal and Infant Care Services. Because of this a national social work licensing exam has been developed in order to ensure parity of quality of licensing criteria among the states. This licensing examination is being used in all states where clinical social workers come under licensing regulations.

Practice Settings

A very high proportion of direct services in counseling and psychotherapy in this country is delivered by clincial social workers, mostly under institutional auspices, but to an increasing degree, privately (Grinnell & Kyte, 1977). Most pertinent for this chapter, social workers are found in increasing numbers to be providing mental health services in outpatient clinics, psychiatric day and night facilities, residential treatment centers for emotionally disturbed children and adults, separate psychiatric services in general hospitals, private psychiatric hospitals, state and county mental hospitals, Veterans Administration psychiatric departments, and other multiservice mental health facilities (Bass & Craven, 1978).

Strengths and Unique Features of Clinical Social Workers

The two particular and unique strengths of clinical social workers are: 1) the use of social planning and community organization skills in effecting change and development in larger population groups; and 2) the use of clinical intervention directed toward development and change in individuals, families, small groups, and the situations that infringe upon them (Cohen, personal communication, 1979).* Clinical social work may be conceptualized as "psychotherapy plus" (Strean, 1978).

If we accept the definition of psychotherapy as a form of professional help that addresses itself to the internal life of the client and seeks to modify maladaptive defenses and increase ego strengths, the clinical social worker, as a psychotherapist, seeks to help the

---

*Professor Jerome Cohen, UCLA. Comments during NASWs' National Invitational Forum on Clinical Social Work. Denver, Colorado, June 7–9.

client discharge feelings and examine behavior and attitudes through the use of a controlled professional relationship. However, the clinical social worker never loses sight of the client's interactions and transactions *within a social context* but seeks to modify those forces in the client's environment that interfere with his personal and interpersonal functioning. The social worker relates to and attempts to modify, when he can, "latent forces within organizations that determine the way people are served or not served" (Strean, 1978, p. 37).

With the development of a specialty in clinical social work, social workers continue to emphasize knowledge and skills in psychological assessment of patients by viewing behavior within a developmental framework with an assessment of adaptive skills. The special focus of social work education on diversity of cultures and on viewing human behavior in the social environment gives social work its particular strength as a profession through its capacity to work with patients of all socioeconomic groups.

Curricula in schools of social work preparing students for clinical social work practice contribute to the special strengths of the specialty. There is a real commitment to transmit both the psychodynamic content and the social content that social work history has repeatedly demonstrated is necessary in order to work with individuals, families, and groups. No other profession in the human services field (except, perhaps, some relatively recent training programs in community psychiatry) aspire to provide the comprehensive social and psychological education that we in clinical social work can offer at our best.

Clinical social work is a logical extension and expansion of social work philosophy articulated many years ago. The strength of clinical social work is demonstrated in the writings of Bertha Reynolds (1934), who stated that "No [therapy] can succeed in isolating a person's attitudes and treating them apart from the conditions of his life in which they find expression" (pp. 126–127). Could any better argument be made for describing the strength of clinical social work as the view of man as a biopsychosocial being?

Weaknesses of Specialty

The diversity, flexibility, and responsiveness to societal needs have resulted in a lack of clarity and specificity about what a clinical social worker is. The profession continues to struggle with how to organize itself in relation to *persons, problems,* and *situations.* Clinical social work is a young profession in terms of common agreement by its members of role and function and is now just beginning to emerge more clearly as a profession with recognizable and accredited skills.

Because we share much in common with other clinical disciplines, distinctive territoriality is difficult to map. We certainly are theory borrowers and are synthesizers and appliers. We have contributed our share of practice theory, but there is a need for more research concerning the effectiveness of treatment approaches.

Finally, there must be careful attention to the length of graduate educational time for clinical social workers: "Clinical excellence requires slow and disciplined seasoning and maturing and under careful tutelage" (Cooper, 1980, p. 27). Journeymen clinicians are not made in two years of study. Nevertheless, the master's level of education can provide solid beginning workers and provide them with adequate preparation for learning either on the job or in extended formal education. More doctoral programs in clinical social work education must be developed, and an expansion of training institutes is necessary.

Interface with Other Core Disciplines

The clinical social worker plays a vital part in the interdisciplinary team. Because of knowledge of the societal context in which the patient/client finds himself, the social worker can provide services, not only as therapist, but also as planner and advocate.

References

Addams, J. *Twenty Years at Hull House.* New York: Macmillan, 1918.
Bartlett, H.M. Toward clarification and improvement of social work practice. *Social Work* 3(2):3–9, 1958.

Bass, R.D. & Craven, R.B. *Manpower issues in community mental health programs (Report, Vol. No. 11. ADAMHA Manpower Policy Analysis Task Force*. Rockville, MD: National Institute of Mental Health, September, 1978.

Berkman, T. *Practice of Social Workers in Psychiatric Hospitals and Clinics*. American Association of Psychiatric Social Workers, Inc., 1953.

Chestang, L.W. Competencies and knowledge in clinical social work: Dual perspective. *National Association of Social Worker's Conference Proceedings—Toward a Definition of Clinical Social Work* (P.L. Ewalt [Ed.]). Washington, DC: National Association of Social Workers, 1979.

Cohen, N. *Social Work in the American Tradition* (pp. 8-10). New York: The Dryden Press, Inc., 1958.

Cooper, S. The masters and beyond, In J. Mishne (Ed.), *Psychotherapy and Training in Clinical Social Work*. New York: Gardner Press, 1980.

Council on Social Work Education. *Statistics on Social Work Education in the United States: 1977*. Unpublished report, 1978.

Education for Psychiatric Social Work: Proceedings of the Dartmouth Conference. Unpublished proceedings distributed by the American Association of Psychiatric Social Workers (now part of the National Association of Social Workers). Silver Springs: MD, 1950.

Grinnell, R.M. Jr., & Kyte, N.S. The future of clinical practice: A study. *Clinical Social Work Journal*, :132-138, 1977.

Hamilton, G. *Theory and Practice of Social Work* (2nd ed., rev.) (p. 6). New York: Columbia University Press, 1951.

Kendall, K. (Ed.). *Social Work Values in an Age of Discontent*. New York: Council of Social Work Education, 1970.

Kubie, L. The retreat from patients. *Archives of General Psychiatry*, 24:98-106, 1971.

Mangold, M.M. (Ed.). *Social Casework* (special issue): *Family Life Today: Critical Issues and Lasting Values*, 57(6), pp. 35-413, 1976.

Minahan, A. Editorial. *Social Work*, :171, 1980.

National Association of Social Workers. *Register of Clinical Social Workers*. Washington, DC: Author, 1976.

Northern, H. *Clinical Social Work*. New York: Columbia University Press, 1982.

Perlman, H.H. Believing and doing: Values in social work education. *Social Casework*, 57(6), p. 382, 1976.

Pinkus, H. et al. [Education at the master's level for the practice of clinical social work]. Unpublished position paper, 1975.

Reynolds, B.C. A study of responsibility in social casework. *Smith College Studies in Social Work*, pp. 126-127, September 1934.

Richmond, M.E. *Social Diagnosis*. New York: Russell Sage Foundation, 1917.

Strean, H.S. *Clinical Social Work: Theory and Practice*. New York: The Free Press, 1978.

Woods, M.E. *The implications of psychosocial practice for clinical social work education*. Paper presented at the Conference on Clinical Social Work, London, England, June, 1981.

Younghusband, E. *Social Work and Social Change*. London: Allen & Unwin, 1964.

APPENDIX C

PSYCHIATRIC/MENTAL HEALTH NURSING

by Shirley A. Smoyak, R.N., Ph.D.

The historical functions of all women—to bathe, to care for, to nurture both the very young and the sick or debilitated and to soothe and comfort people generally—were transferred in part in modern times from homes to hospitals. It is in this sense that every woman thinks of herself as a "nurse." It also accounts for society's reluctance to be serious about academic education for nurses (Peplau, 1977). Women were expected to know nursing without education: "Nursing, as an occupation, developed out of the social need for care of the sick" (Peplau, 1977, p. 43). In the past century it has been tranformed from a largely pragmatic, general practice of all women to an academically based profession having highly specialized areas. This appendix addresses one specialty in nursing—psychiatric or mental health nursing.

Basic Tenets

Mental health care is a subunit of comprehensive health care, which is an intricate complex of services to individuals, families, and society. Nursing encompasses promotion and maintenance of health; prevention, detection, and treatment of responses to trauma and illness; and restoration to the highest possible levels of health. Nurses recognize that there is a high degree of interdependence

Shirley A. Smoyak, R.N., Ph.D., is Professor, School of Nursing, Rutgers University, New Brunswick, NJ.

inherent in health care among the elements of service, in relationships among professional groups, and with the public: "Nursing contributes to virtually all aspects of the health care delivery system, inclusive of those services identified as mental health" (American Nurses' Association [ANA], 1976, p. 1). "The profession is committed to health and to the fullest possible utilization of human potential" (ANA, 1976b, p. 1). Nurses feel a responsibility to act as advocates for the public and have acted to facilitate changes in health care systems such that fragmentation and maldistribution of resources are minimized. "Continuing evidence of unresolved problems, especially in environmental conditions and discontinuities in service which violated human dignity, impel nurses to work more effectively as consumer advocates" (ANA, 1976b, p. 1).

As professional persons, nurses assume they are accountable for their actions and insist on the right to determine the dimensions of their practice in an autonomous fashion. While desiring that the public be protected, they insist that nurses define the legitimate scope of their authority and expertise. Through academic "gatekeepers," professional certification, peer review and state boards of nursing, nurses control access to the professional ranks, judging and monitoring the competence to practice nursing.

Psychiatric nurses, as well as the other specialty groups, practice nursing by adhering to the *Code for Nurses,* which provides guidance for conduct and relationships in carrying out nursing responsibilities consistent with the ethical obligations of the profession and quality of nursing care (ANA, 1976a). Synoptically, the code states that nurses respect human dignity, safeguard clients' privacy, protect patients from illegal or harmful practitioners, remain competent, exercise informed judgement, contribute to the development of the profession, and collaborate with members of the health professions in meeting health needs of the public.

> Psychiatric and mental health nursing, like all other specialties in nursing, has discrete as well as shared functions for which it is responsible to society. The major distinguishing characteristics of psychiatric and mental health nursing prac-

tice derive from the synthesis of knowledge and experience in both nursing and mental health. Aspects of nursing which support the distinctive contributions of nurses to comprehensive mental health care include:

1. Nursing's commitment to holistic and continuous personal care of individuals, founded on theory and clinical practice, which utilizes content from the social, biological, and physical sciences;
2. Nursing's primary focus on helping persons attain their highest possible level of health, which includes but transcends traditional illness orientation;
3. Nursing's integration of content and experience related to both the medical and social systems models in the conduct of its clinical practice and research;
4. The use of the nursing process as the dominant modality, involving systematic and identifiable steps which must be accounted for, professionally, in terms of quality. (ANA, 1976b, p. 2)

Psychiatric and mental health nurses practice largely in collaboration and coordination with a variety of other professions, working with and on behalf of the client. Overlapping of roles and shared functions create tensions and potential for conflict, which requires that nurses and their colleagues address the jurisdictional issues calmly, respectfully, and often. Nurses believe that interprofessional planning and evaluation of services contribute effectively to high quality of care.

Functional Definition

Psychiatric and mental health nursing is a specialized area of nursing practice employing theories of human behavior as its science and purposeful use of self as its art. It is directed toward both preventive and corrective impacts upon mental disorders and their sequelae and is concerned with the promotion of optimal mental health for society, the community, and those individuals who live within it. (ANA, 1976b, p. 2)

The practice of psychiatric and mental health nursing is characterized by those aspects of clinical nursing care that involve interpersonal relationships with individuals and groups, as well as a variety of other activities. These activities include (ANA, 1976b):

1. Providing a therapeutic milieu, concerned largely with the sociopsychological aspects of clients' environments.
2. Working with clients concerning the here-and-now living problems they confront.
3. Accepting and using the surrogate parent role.
4. Detecting and caring for somatic aspects of clients' health problems, including responses to drugs and other treatments.
5. Teaching with specific reference to emotional health as evidenced by various behavioral patterns.
6. Assuming the role of social agent concerned with improvement of recreational, occupational, and social competence.
7. Providing leadership and clinical assistance to other nursing personnel and generic health care workers.
8. Conducting psychotherapy.
9. Engaging in social and community action roles related to mental health.

Psychiatric and mental health nurses use selected theoretical frameworks, with particular emphasis on the psychosocial and biophysical sciences. While theory of human behavior and concern for psychosocial and cultural aspects of health and illness are an integral part of all nursing practice, the specialty area of psychiatric and mental health nursing is characterized by a greater amount and depth of such knowledge and specialized competence in its application. The nurses' flexible use of different types of theory, pertinent to both the medical and sociocultural models of mental health and illness, facilitates comprehensive, balanced perceptions of and responses to clients' problems in light of nurses' purposes and the setting.

Some examples of particular theoretical sources commonly used by psychiatric/mental health nurses include: systems theory; symbolic interactionism; communication, somatic, psychopharmacological, learning, psychoanalytic, stress, and crisis theories. An additional and essential body of knowledge for practice rests in the scholarly conceptualizations of psychiatric nursing practice and in research findings generated from intra- and cross-disciplinary studies of other nurses.

Training

There are two types of practitioners in psychiatric and mental health settings: one is a psychiatric or mental health nurse and the other a clinical specialist in psychiatric or mental health nursing. The former is prepared at the baccalaureate level and the latter at the master's level, generally in a program that emphasizes a clinical practicum of roughly 12 to 20 hours per week over two academic years. At this point in time there are still large numbers of nurses working in psychiatric facilities who are prepared only by a hospital diploma program or an associate of arts degree. The basic academic requirement for entry into professional nursing practice is the baccalaureate degree.

The clinical specialist (with a master's degree) is distinguished by in-depth command of knowledge about psychosocial theories of human behavior, supervised clinical experience, and skill in the application of theory in the practice of individual, group, or family therapy. Doctoral education in psychiatric and mental health nursing is now pursued by a substantial number of nurses. These programs at the doctoral level emphasize 1) research and theory development in the science of psychiatric and mental health nursing; or 2) advance development of the nurse-therapist role with the research component directed toward the investigation of specific clinical problems. The first type of program, the traditional research-oriented focus, generally leads to a Ph.D. degree, whereas the second usually leads to a D.N.S. degree. Nurses prepared at the doctoral level from both types of programs contribute to the advancement of knowledge in the field of psychiatric and mental health nursing through research and scholarship.

Psychiatric and mental health nurses function in different settings and work with a variety of patients or client populations. Each of these settings or populations may be used to define a subspecialty within the general field of psychiatric and mental health nursing. Three major subspecialty areas are defined in terms of the age of the client: 1) child, 2) adult, and 3) gerontological psychiatric and mental health nursing. Generally, clinical specialists have chosen to define themselves as either child psychiatric and mental health nurses or adult psychiatric and mental health nurses: however, many clinical specialists find that by using family therapy they can be more effective, as they are working with the entire range of age groups within a family. Gerontological psychiatric and mental health nursing is an emerging subspecialty area. Preparation at the graduate level is available in each of these three subspecialty areas.

Certification

Through the Division of Psychiatric and Mental Health Nursing of the American Nurses' Association, a nurse may be certified at either the generalist or specialist level. Certification requires sitting for an examination and, at the specialist level, producing documentation of one's clinical practice, analysis of selected case studies, and evidence of supervision. The certification examination at the master's level is specific to age groups and modalities of practice.

Sites for Practice

Psychiatric nurses practice in a variety of settings, ranging from institutions characterized by intense teamwork and high technology to more loosely organized agencies. Patient care settings include primary, secondary, and tertiary categories and span the gamut from proprietary types to all levels of government (city, county, state, federal).

The term "setting" refers to more than the physical surroundings or milieu of a clinical facility. It implies the aggregate of both the physical arrangements and those philosophical influences that give a practice environment special character. The total of the emotional climate, ideology, conventions of governance and finances, and purposes, whether planned or implicit, are included.

> Two principal arrangements for the clinical practice of psychi-
> atric and mental health nursing are: organized settings and
> self-employment. Nurses who work within organized settings
> are remunerated for their services on either a salaried or
> fee-for-service basis. These settings are largely shaped by
> administrative policies which either foster or limit the full
> utilization of the nurse's capabilities. A growing number of
> psychiatric and mental health nursing specialists are self-
> employed, realizing reimbursement for their services through
> third-party payments and direct client fees. Some of these
> specialists maintain staff privileges with insititutional facili-
> ties. (ANA, 1976b, p. 7)

Strengths of the Specialty

The primary strength of the specialty in nursing, psychiatric/mental health nursing, is that its clinical practice is firmly based upon theoretical frameworks and models. Other areas of nursing, because of historical developments, tend to be more pragmatic or guided by principles as opposed to theories. Psychiatric nursing, instead, is clearly committed to understanding the phenomena of disturbances in human behavior and using applications of theory to guide intervention strategies. Psychiatric nurses are taught to be exceptional observers, to record these observations, and then to use them to determine the appropriate, theory-guided intervention. Astute nurses rely on the analysis of the situation as a practice guide; they tend to be more thoughtful than to operate in an ad hoc manner.

Psychiatric nurses have a firm foundation in biological and somatic theories and research, as well as in the psychological and sociocultural dimensions. They are able to determine whether or not a given behavioral disturbance might have organic underpinnings. Because they operate from the broad scope of a holistic perspective, they do remember in their day-to-day practice that the head is connected to the body and that one influences the other greatly. A mentally healthy outlook is easier to achieve in an organically healthy body. Nurses remind their clients about the benefits of paying attention to their physiological as well as their psychosocial selves. Many psychiatric nurses have been prepared to do basic physical examinations and health assessments. Particularly in areas where access to comprehensive health care in unevenly distributed, psychiatric nurses provide a much-needed service. Because nurses are well versed in the physiological as well as the psychosocial aspects of human body processes, they are looked upon as resources for information about nutrition, exercise, immunization, special diets, and so on. They provide assessments for both the family member under treatment, as well as others, to separate the normal from the not-normal in any body system.

The secondary socialization to the profession, nursing, has historical roots of producing in its recruits a firm foundation of a sense of responsibility to patients and families and a respect for life. Nurses need not be reminded constantly to "do no harm." They have internalized a sense of being accountable for their actions within the scope of their clinical abilities.

Again, as an outcome of their secondary socialization to the profession, nurses are resourceful, innovative, creative practitioners. They learn very early in their training to do without or to use what is available to "make do." Their training in public health environments and in patients' homes, of all social classes, enhances this resourcefulness. Very often, in the middle of the night or on weekends, they are the only resource within hospitals and must, therefore, creatively and effectively handle the whole range of human behavior from violent outbursts to withdrawals and suicide attempts. Their preventive and interventive actions are relied upon by patients and other mental health staff on a 24-hour, seven-day-a-week basis.

While well prepared in a broad, holistic way, nurses do not

characteristically leap ahead into territories that they do not know. They have a realistic sense of their limitations, based on the scope of their education. They are very ready to say what they know, as well as what they do not know, and to consult, refer, cooperate, collaborate, or seek more personal knowledge, as is appropriate in each situation. They are not likely to see themselves as all-knowing or omnipotent and not likely to endanger patients by experimental or ill-founded approaches. Part of the reason that nurses are sued less often than their colleagues rests in the felt assurance and comfort of their patients that the care they have received has been safe and humane.

Because nurses, in their generic preparation as generalists, have worked with patients whose illnesses or incapacities are of long duration and tending toward high recidivism (alcoholism, arthritis), they develop a patience and a respect for time (duration of illness), and that is greatly appreciated by their patients. Nurses are able to judge when a patient in a rehabilitation program for a chronic condition needs a little bit more time or a well-aimed push. Waiting for a patient to become ready is not seen as a waste of time but an opportunity to establish better rapport and for application of readying approaches.

Nurses frequently use a general systems approach and include all family members in their assessment and treatment plans. They are not likely to interpret symptoms as "belonging" to individual clients but rather to define them as signals of system distress.

Nurses are willing to go to the patient or family and to meet and treat them in their own settings. Smoyak (1977) has described the benefits of such an approach in a chapter, "Homes: A Natural Environment for Family Therapy." This approach provides a far more accurate data base about pathological processes, especially in light of more recent theories, and its advantages far outweigh any associated costs.

Weakness of the Specialty

Most nurses are women and, unfortunately, the positive effects of the women's movement have not yet erased the tendencies toward dependence, subservience, and obsequiousness which so badly hamper the profession. Some nurses still downplay their knowledge and hide their bright lights under the proverbial bushels. They rarely "toot their own horns." The nurse assumes that if she discovers something, clinically, it is not really new and others have known it before. Nurses tend to believe that their uncommon findings are someone else's common knowledge.

Certainly nurses today are more assertive than they were 20 years ago, but the damages to their self-esteem, historically, have been considerable. They are still somewhat reluctant to use their authority, based on education, license, and social mandate, to act individually and collectively to create change.

Too many nurses see what they do as "work" or a "job" rather than view themselves as career-oriented professionals. This tendency has several very deleterious spinoffs—not pursuing further education, not engaging in research, not writing or publishing the results of their clinical work, and not becoming organizationally involved in professional politics. Because they are less likely to be career-minded, they often lack a professional mentor to guide their way. Ironically, they tend to provide guiding services to others (traditionally, nurses taught and supervised aids and assistants in all psychiatric settings) but do not seek guides or mentors for themselves.

Until recently, nurses tended to seek the advice or consultation of nonnurses (e.g., psychiatrists, psychologists) rather than to rely on the knowledge and expertise of other nurses. They valued the ideas and products of men rather than women. The tide is beginning to turn, and the new sense of professional self-worth is leading nurses to seek other nurses for clinical dialogue.

In underselling themselves, psychiatric nurses have tended to produce a kind of "deflation" among all mental health professions. If a nurse working in a CMHC collects less than what she's worth, the income of others will also be affected.

Nurses have become much more cognitive in their clinical approaches to psychiatric patients, but they still tend to use "radar" or an ill-defined or ill-described method to sense something is wrong on a unit or with a particular patient. Until they are able to translate these right-brain talents into speech, it will be difficult at best, and more likely impossible, to teach these "early warning" signal detection skills to others.

There is great variability in the educational preparation of psychiatric nurses. Some have very well-grounded clinical practice in their backgrounds; others do not. Psychopharmacology is often overlooked or treated superficially in the curriculum. There is no national consensus, encouraged by an academic accreditation process, which sets guidelines for theories and clinical strategies to be included.

Unique Characteristics of the Specialty

The nurse is the member of the mental health care team who has the responsibility for the continuity of patient care in inpatient settings and the integration of a myriad of services in outpatient settings. Within hospitals they diagnose and monitor the milieu in which patients are treated. They are responsible for the physical as well as the psychosocial environments.

They are in charge of transitions. They orient patients upon admission, integrate their within-hospital shifts and changes, prepare them for discharge and follow them, frequently, into the community. A new subspecialty of psychiatric nursing is liaison nursing. These clinical specialists provide consultation about psychiatric and behavioral problems to staff nurses in general hospital units and to public health nurses in communities.

While all four of the core mental health professions share roughly the same body of knowledge, the psychiatric nurse is unique in the following respects:

1. Uses biological as well as psychosocial theories in providing holistic health care;
2. Provides continuity of patient care on all shifts and days;
3. Plans, monitors, and executes transitions for patients among modalities, services, and settings; and
4. Defines the jurisdiction of her practice to be the diagnosis and treatment of human responses to actual or potential health problems.

Nurses are close to their patients, both physically and emotionally. They frequently touch them in the course of providing care. The tremendous impact of something so simple as touching has recently been documented by the research of two nurses (Duffy & Steuding, 1982). In separate studies in a long-term care facility, these psychiatric nurses discovered that patients who were touched more frequently by staff were less angry, depressed, and hostile than those who were touched less frequently.

Evaluation and/or Outcome Data

Psychiatric nurses have been very remiss in conducting the type of research that yields definitive outcome data. It is impossible to document scientifically, at this point in time, that psychiatric nurses do make a difference in terms of patient outcomes. Because of the tendency in mental health to work in teams, a further difficulty is research design. With two or more clinicians collaborating on a given case or with a family, it cannot be demonstrated that one professional was more effective or more useful to the client than another. The confounding of results in such situations is profound.

What is needed, however, is another kind of documentation. Given the push toward rapid return to the community, philosophical and ethical questions can be raised concerning the human dilemma of the clients who lack continuity of care. How do nurses practice differently under these rapid changes? What accommodations in therapeutic approaches are being made to give service to the new chronic (never institutionalized) population?

Psychiatric nurses have served, in the past, as mentors for nonnurses. Unfortunately, their influence over the career development of others has never been systematically studied.

Relationship with the Other Core Disciplines

The Joint Commission on Interprofessional Affairs (JCIA) was founded in 1975. The members are representatives of the American Nurses' Association, the American Psychiatric Association, the American Psychological Association, and the National Association of Social Workers. The Commission was convened after one organization critically commented about another organization in testimony before the United States Congress. Following this commentary, the organizational leaders realized the destructiveness of fighting and created the JCIA.

Each organization has three representatives, two appointed members, and one assigned staff person. The Commission meets three times a year to discuss legislation, reimbursement, education, and patient care. The goal is to achieve interprofessional trust and cooperation rather than divisiveness and animosity. Gradually, the Commission has learned to work together, having overcome the initial caution, suspicion, and parochialism. JCIA has recognized that it is too easy for organizations with legitimate differences of opinion, policy, or goals to develop an unnecessarily destructive attitude and approach toward each other. In recognition of this, the Commission has strongly recommended that the participating organizations adopt common guidelines on interprofessional ethics. Implementation of such guidelines will help to eliminate inaccurate statements, accusations, and animosities and lead toward a more collaborative relationship.

References

American Nurses' Association. *Code for Nurses with Interpretive Statements* (adopted 1950 and periodically revised). (ANA Publication No. G-56) 1976 Kansas City, MO: ANA Division on Psychiatric and Mental Health Nursing Practice, 1976a.

American Nurses' Association. *Statement of Psychiatric and Mental Health Nursing Practice,* Kansas City, MO: ANA Division on Psychiatric and Mental Health Nursing Practice, 1976b.

Duffy, E. & Steuding, E. *An Exploratory Study: The Effects of Touch on the Elderly in a Nursing Home.* Unpublished master's thesis, Rutgers University, New Brunswick, NJ, 1982.

Peplau, H.E. The changing view of nursing. *International Nursing Review,* 24(2)43-45, 1977.

Smoyak, S. Homes: A natural environment for family therapy. In J. Hall & B. Weaver (Eds.), *Distributive Nursing Practice: A Systems Approach to Community Health* (pp. 369-380). New York: J.B. Lippincott Co., 1977.

NAME INDEX

SUBJECT INDEX

GAP COMMITTEES AND MEMBERSHIP

COMMITTEE ON ADOLESCENCE
Clarice J. Kestenbaum, New York, N.Y.,
 Chairperson
Hector R. Bird, Santurce, P.R.
Ian A. Canino, New York, N.Y.
Warren J. Gadpaille, Denver, Colo.
Michael G. Kalogerakis, New York,
 N.Y.
Silvio J. Onesti, Jr., Belmont, Mass.

COMMITTEE ON AGING
Gene D. Cohen, Rockville, Md.,
 Chairperson
Eric D. Caine, Rochester, N.Y.
Charles M. Gaitz, Houston, Tex.
Gabe J. Maletta, Minneapolis, Minn.
Robert J. Nathan, Philadelphia, Pa.
George H. Pollock, Chicago, Ill.
Kenneth M. Sakauye, Chicago, Ill.
Charles A. Shamoian, White Plains,
 N.Y.
F. Conyers Thompson, Jr., Atlanta, Ga.

COMMITTEE ON ALCOHOLISM AND THE
 ADDICTIONS
Edward J. Khantzian, Haverhill, Mass.,
 Chairperson
Richard J. Frances, Newark, N.J.
Sheldon I. Miller, Newark, N.J.
Robert B. Millman, New York, N.Y.
Steven M. Mirin, Westwood, Mass.
Edgar P. Nace, Dallas, Tex.
Norman L. Paul, Lexington, Mass.

COMMITTEE ON CHILD PSYCHIATRY
Theodore Shapiro, New York, N.Y.,
 Chairperson
James M. Bell, Canaan, N.Y.
Harlow Donald Dunton, New York,
 N.Y.
Joseph Fischhoff, Detroit, Mich.
John F. McDermott, Jr., Honolulu,
 Hawaii
John Schowalter, New Haven, Conn.
Peter E. Tanguay, Los Angeles, Calif.
Lenore Terr, San Francisco, Calif.

COMMITTEE ON COLLEGE STUDENTS
Myron B. Liptzin, Chapel Hill, N.C.,
 Chairperson
Robert L. Arnstein, Hamden, Conn.
Varda Backus, La Jolla, Calif.
Harrison P. Eddy, New York, N.Y.
Malkah Tolpin Notman, Brookline,
 Mass.
Gloria C. Onque, Pittsburgh, Pa.
Elizabeth Aub Reid, Cambridge,
 Mass.
Earle Silber, Chevy Chase, Md.
Tom G. Stauffer, White Plains, N.Y.

COMMITTEE ON CULTURAL PSYCHIATRY
Ezra E.H. Griffith, New Haven, Conn.,
 Chairperson
Edward F. Foulks, New Orleans, La.
Pedro Ruiz, Houston, Tex.
John P. Spiegel, Waltham, Mass.

Ronald M. Wintrob, Providence, R.I.
Joe Yamamoto, Los Angeles, Calif.

COMMITTEE ON THE FAMILY
W. Robert Beavers, Dallas, Tex.,
    Chairperson
Ellen M. Berman, Merrion, Pa.
Lee Combrinck-Graham, Evanston,
    Ill.
Ira D. Glick, New York, N.Y.
Frederick Gottlieb, Los Angeles, Calif.
Henry U. Grunebaum, Cambridge,
    Mass.
Herta A. Guttman, Montreal, Quebec
Judith Landau-Stanton, Rochester,
    N.Y.
Ann L. Price, Hartford, Conn.
Lyman C. Wynne, Rochester, N.Y.

COMMITTEE ON HANDICAPS
Norman R. Bernstein, Cambridge,
    Mass.,
    Chairperson
Meyer S. Gunther, Chicago, Ill.
William H. Sack, Portland, Oreg.
William A. Sonis, Minneapolis, Minn.
George Tarjan, Los Angeles, Calif.
Thomas G. Webster, Washington, D.C.
Henry H. Work, Bethesda, Md.

COMMITTEE ON HUMAN SEXUALITY
Bertram H. Schaffner, New York, N.Y.,
    Chairperson
Paul L. Adams, Galveston, Tex.
Johanna A. Hoffman, Scottsdale, Ariz.

COMMITTEE ON INTERNATIONAL
    RELATIONS
Vamik D. Volkan, Charlottesville, Va.,
    Chairperson
Francis F. Barnes, Chevy Chase, Md.
Robert M. Dorn, El Macero, Calif.

John S. Kafka, Washington, D.C.
Otto F. Kernberg, White Plains, N.Y.
John E. Mack, Chestnut Hill, Mass.
Rita R. Rogers, Palos Verdes Estates,
    Calif.
Stephen B. Shanfield, San Antonio,
    Tex.

COMMITTEE ON MEDICAL EDUCATION
David R. Hawkins, Chicago, Ill.,
    Chairperson
Gene Abroms, Ardmore, Pa.
Charles M. Culver, Hanover, N.H.
Steven L. Dubovsky, Denver, Colo.
Saul I. Harrison, Torrance, Calif.
Harold I. Lief, Philadelphia, Pa.
Carol Nadelson, Boston, Mass.
Carolyn B. Robinowitz, Washington,
    D.C.
Stephen C. Scheiber, Evanston, Ill.
Sidney L. Werkman, Denver, Colo.
Veva H. Zimmerman, New York, N.Y.

COMMITTEE ON MENTAL HEALTH
    SERVICES
Jose Maria Santiago, Tucson, Ariz.,
    Chairperson
John M. Hamilton, Baltimore, Md.
W. Walter Menninger, Topeka, Kans.
Steven S. Sharfstein, Baltimore, Md.
Herzl R. Spiro, Milwaukee, Wis.
William L. Webb, Jr., Hartford, Conn.
George F. Wilson, Somerville, N.J.
Jack A. Wolford, Pittsburgh, Pa.

COMMITTEE ON PLANNING AND
    MARKETING
Robert W. Gibson, Towson, Md.,
    Chairperson
Allan Beigel, Tucson, Ariz.
Doyle I. Carson, Dallas, Tex.
Harvey L. Ruben, New Haven,
    Conn.

Melvin Sabshin, Washington, D.C.
Michael R. Zales, Greenwich, Conn.

COMMITTEE ON PREVENTIVE PSYCHIATRY
Stephen Fleck, New Haven, Conn.,
Chairperson
Viola W. Bernard, New York, N.Y.
Stanley I. Greenspan, Bethesda, Md.
William H. Hetznecker, Philadelphia,
Pa.
Harris B. Peck, New Rochelle, N.Y.
Naomi Rae-Grant, Hamilton, Ontario
Anne Marie Wolf-Schatz, Philadelphia,
Pa.
Morton M. Silverman, Rockville, Md.

COMMITTEE ON PSYCHIATRY AND THE
COMMUNITY
Kenneth Minkoff, Woburn, Mass.,
Chairperson
C. Knight Aldrich, Charlottesville, Va.
David G. Greenfeld, New Haven, Conn.
H. Richard Lamb, Los Angeles, Calif.
John C. Nemiah, Hanover, N.H.
Rebecca L. Potter, Tucson, Ariz.
Alexander S. Rogawski, Los Angeles,
Calif.
John J. Schwab, Louisville, Ky.
John A. Talbott, Baltimore, Md.
Charles B. Wilkinson, Kansas City, Mo.

COMMITTEE ON PSYCHIATRY AND LAW
Jonas R. Rappeport, Baltimore, Md.,
Chairperson
Park E. Dietz, Charlottesville, Va.
John Donnelly, Hartford, Conn.
Carl P. Malmquist, Minneapolis, Minn.
Herbert C. Modlin, Topeka, Kans.
Phillip J. Resnick, Cleveland, Ohio
Loren J. Roth, Pittsburgh, Pa.
Joseph Satten, San Francisco, Calif.
William D. Weitzel, Lexington, Ky.
Howard V. Zonana, New Haven, Conn.

COMMITTEE ON PSYCHIATRY AND
RELIGION
Albert J. Lubin, Woodside, Calif.,
Chairperson
Sidney Furst, Bronx, N.Y.
Richard C. Lewis, New Haven, Conn.
Earl A. Loomis, Jr., Augusta, Ga.
Abigail R. Ostow, Cambridge, Mass.
Mortimer Ostow, Bronx, N.Y.
Sally K. Severino, White Plains, N.Y.
Clyde R. Snyder, Fayetteville, N.C.

COMMITTEE ON PSYCHIATRY IN INDUSTRY
Barrie S. Greiff, Cambridge, Mass.,
Chairperson
Peter L. Brill, Philadelphia, Pa.
Duane Q. Hagen, St. Louis, Mo.
R. Edward Huffman, Asheville, N.C.
David E. Morrison, Palatine, Ill.
David B. Robbins, Chappaqua, N.Y.
Jay B. Rohrlich, New York, N.Y.
Clarence J. Rowe, St. Paul, Minn.
Jeffrey L. Speller, Alexandria, Va.

COMMITTEE ON PSYCHOPATHOLOGY
David A. Adler, Boston, Mass.,
Chairperson
Jeffrey Berlant, Summit, N.J.
Robert E. Drake, Hanover, N.H.
James J. Ellison, Watertown, Mass.
Howard H. Goldman, Rockville, Md.
Richard E. Renneker, Los Angeles,
Calif.

COMMITTEE ON PUBLIC EDUCATION
Keith H. Johansen, Dallas, Tex.,
Chairperson
Susan J. Blumenthal, Washington, D.C.
Robert J. Campbell, New York, N.Y.
Steven E. Katz, New York, N.Y.
Robert A. Solow, Beverly Hills, Calif.
Kenneth N. Vogtsberger, San Antonio,
Tex.

COMMITTEE ON RESEARCH
Robert Cancro, New York, N.Y.,
    Chairperson
Kenneth Z. Altshuler, Dallas, Tex.
Jack A. Grebb, New York, N.Y.
John H. Greist, Madison, Wisc.
Jerry M. Lewis, Dallas, Tex.
Morris A. Lipton, Chapel Hill, N.C.
John G. Looney, Durham, N.C.
Sidney Malitz, New York, N.Y.
Zebulon Taintor, Orangeburg, N.Y.

COMMITTEE ON SOCIAL ISSUES
Ian E. Alger, New York, N.Y.,
    Chairperson
William R. Beardslee, Boston, Mass.
Paul J. Fink, Philadelphia, Pa.
Judith H. Gold, Halifax, Nova Scotia
Roderic Gorney, Los Angeles, Calif.
Martha J. Kirkpatrick, Los Angeles,
    Calif.
Perry Ottenberg, Philadelphia, Pa.
Kendon W. Smith, Piermont, N.Y.

COMMITTEE ON THERAPEUTIC CARE
Milton Kramer, Cincinnati, Ohio,
    Chairperson
Bernard Bandler, Cambridge, Mass.
Thomas E. Curtis, Chapel Hill, N.C.
Donald W. Hammersley, Washington,
    D.C.
William B. Hunter, III, Albuquerque,
    N.M.
Roberto L. Jimenez, San Antonio, Tex.
William W. Richards, Anchorage,
    Alaska

COMMITTEE ON THERAPY
Allen D. Rosenblatt, La Jolla, Calif.,
    Chairperson
Jules R. Bemporad, Boston, Mass.
Henry W. Brosin, Tucson, Ariz.
Eugene B. Feigelson, Brooklyn, N.Y.

Robert Michels, New York, N.Y.
Andrew P. Morrison, Cambridge,
    Mass.
William C. Offenkrantz, Milwaukee,
    Wis.

CONTRIBUTING MEMBERS
John E. Adams, Gainesville, Fl.
Carlos C. Alden, Jr., Buffalo, N.Y.

Eric A. Baum, Sarasota, Fl.
Spencer Bayles, Houston, Tex.
C. Christian Beels, New York, N.Y.
Elissa P. Benedek, Ann Arbor, Mich.
Sidney Berman, Washington, D.C.
Wilfred Bloomberg, Cambridge, Mass.
H. Keith H. Brodie, Durham, N.C.
Charles M. Bryant, San Francisco,
    Calif.
Ewald W. Busse, Durham, N.C.
Robert N. Butler, New York, N.Y.

Eugene M. Caffey Jr., Bowie, Md.
Ian L.W. Clancey, Ontario, Canada
Sanford I. Cohen, Boston, Mass.

James S. Eaton, Jr., Washington, D.C.
Lloyd C. Elam, Nashville, Tenn.
Stanley H. Eldred, Belmont, Mass.
Joseph T. English, New York, N.Y.
Louis C. English, Pomona, N.Y.

Sherman C. Feinstein, Highland Park,
    Ill.
Archie R. Foley, New York, N.Y.
Daniel X. Freedman, Los Angeles,
    Calif.

Henry J. Gault, Highland Park, Ill.
Alexander Gralnick, Port Chester, N.Y.
Joseph M. Green, Madison, Wis.
Milton Greenblatt, Sepulveda, Calif.
Lawrence F. Greenleigh, Los Angeles,
    Calif.
Jon E. Gudeman, Lexington, Mass.

Seymour L. Halleck, Chapel Hill, N.C.
Stanley Hammons, Lexington, Ky.
J. Cotter Hirschberg, Topeka, Kans.

Jay Katz, New Haven, Conn.
James A. Knight, New Orleans, La.
Othilda M. Krug, Cincinnati, Ohio

Alan I. Levenson, Tucson, Ariz.
Ruth W. Lidz, Woodbridge, Conn.
Orlando B. Lightfoot, Boston, Mass.
Reginald S. Lourie, Chevy Chase, Md.
Norman L. Loux, Sellersville, Pa.

John A. MacLeod, Cincinnati, Ohio
Leo Madow, Philadelphia, Pa.
Charles A. Malone, Cleveland, Ohio
Peter A. Martin, Lake Orion, Mich.
Ake Mattsson, Danderyd, Sweden
Alan A. McLean, Westport, Conn.
David Mendell, Houston, Tex.
Roy W. Menninger, Topeka, Kans.
Mary E. Mercer, Nyack, N.Y.
Derek Miller, Chicago, Ill.
Richard D. Morrill, Boston, Mass.

Joseph D. Noshpitz, Washington, D.C.

Bernard L. Pacella, New York, N.Y.
Herbert Pardes, New York, N.Y.
Marvin E. Perkins, Salem, Va.
Betty J. Pfefferbaum, Houston, Tex.

David N. Ratnavale, Bethesda, Md.
Kent E. Robinson, Towson, Md.
Milton Rosenblatt, Sylmar, Calif.
W. Donald Ross, Cincinnati, Ohio
Lester H. Rudy, Chicago, Ill.
George E. Ruff, Philadelphia, Pa.

David S. Sanders, Los Angeles, Calif.
Donald J. Scherl, Brooklyn, N.Y.
Kurt O. Schlesinger, San Francisco,
  Calif.
Charles Shagrass, Philadelphia, Pa.
Miles F. Shore, Boston, Mass.

Albert J. Silverman, Ann Arbor, Mich.
Benson R. Snyder, Cambridge, Mass.
David A. Soskis, Bala Cynwyd, Pa.
Jeanne Spurlock, Washington, D.C.
Brandt F. Steele, Denver, Colo.
Alan A. Stone, Cambridge, Mass.
Robert E. Switzer, Dunn Loring, Va.

Perry C. Talkington, Dallas, Tex.
Bryce Templeton, Philadelphia, Pa.
Prescott W. Thompson, Beaverton,
  Oreg.
Joe P. Tupin, Sacramento, Calif.
John A. Turner, San Francisco, Calif.

Gene L. Usdin, New Orleans, La.

Warren T. Vaughan, Jr., Portola Valley,
  Calif.

Andrew S. Watson, Ann Arbor, Mich.
Joseph B. Wheelwright, Kentfield,
  Calif.
Robert L. Williams, Houston, Tex.
Paul Tyler Wilson, Bethesda, Md.
Sherwyn M. Woods, Los Angeles,
  Calif.

Kent A. Zimmerman, Berkeley, Calif.
Israel Zwerling, Philadelphia, Pa.

LIFE MEMBERS
C. Knight Aldrich, Charlottesville, Va.
Bernard Bandler, Cambridge, Mass.
Walter E. Barton, Hartland, Vt.
Viola W. Bernard, New York, N.Y.
Wilfred Bloomberg, Cambridge, Mass.
Murray Bowen, Chevy Chase, Md.
Henry W. Brosin, Tucson, Ariz.
John Donnelly, Hartford, Conn.
Merrill T. Eaton, Omaha, Neb.
O. Spurgeon English, Narberth, Pa.
Stephen Fleck, New Haven, Conn.
Jerome Frank, Baltimore, Md.
Robert S. Garber, Osprey, Fl.
Robert W. Gibson, Towson, Md.

Paul E. Huston, Iowa City, Iowa
Margaret M. Lawrence, Pomona, N.Y.
Harold I. Lief, Philadelphia, Pa.
Morris A. Lipton, Chapel Hill, N.C.
Judd Marmor, Los Angeles, Calif.
Karl A. Menninger, Topeka, Kans.
Herbert C. Modlin, Topeka, Kans.
John C. Nemiah, Hanover, N.H.
Mabel Ross, Sun City, Ariz.
Julius Schreiber, Washington, D.C.
George Tarjan, Los Angeles, Calif.
Jack A. Wolford, Pittsburgh, Pa.
Henry H. Work, Bethesda, Md.

BOARD OF DIRECTORS

OFFICERS

President
Jerry M. Lewis
Timberlawn Foundation
P.O. Box 270789
Dallas, Tex. 75227

President-Elect
Carolyn B. Robinowitz
Deputy Medical Director for Education
American Psychiatric Association
1400 K Street, N.W.
Washington, D.C. 20005

Secretary
Allan Beigel
30 Camino Español
Tucson, Ariz. 85716

Treasurer
Charles B. Wilkinson
600 E. 22nd Street
Kansas City, Mo. 64108

Board Members
David R. Hawkins
Silvio J. Onesti
John A. Talbott
Lenore Terr

Past Presidents

*William C. Menninger	1946–51
Jack R. Ewalt	1951–53
Walter E. Barton	1953–55
*Sol W. Ginsburg	1955–57
*Dana L. Farnsworth	1957–59
*Marion E. Kenworthy	1959–61
Henry W. Brosin	1961–63
*Leo H. Bartemeier	1963–65
Robert S. Garber	1965–67
Herbert C. Modlin	1967–69
John Donnelly	1969–71
George Tarjan	1971–73
Judd Marmor	1973–75
John C. Nemiah	1975–77
Jack A. Wolford	1977–79
Robert W. Gibson	1979–81
*Jack Weinberg	1981–82
Henry H. Work	1982–85
Michael R. Zales	1985–87

PUBLICATIONS BOARD

Chairman
Alexander S. Rogawski
11665 West Olympic Blvd.
Apt. #302
Los Angeles, Calif. 90064

Robert L. Arnstein
Stanley I. Greenspan
Milton Kramer
W. Walter Menninger
Robert A. Solow

Consultant
John C. Nemiah

Ex-Officio
Jerry M. Lewis
Carolyn B. Robinowitz

_____

* deceased

CONTRIBUTORS
Abbott Laboratories
American Charitable Fund
Dr. and Mrs. Richard Aron
Mr. Robert C. Baker
Maurice Falk Medical Fund
Mrs. Carol Gold
Grove Foundation, Inc.
Miss Gayle Groves
Ittleson Foundation, Inc.
Mr. Barry Jacobson
Mrs. Allan H. Kalmus
Marion E. Kenworthy—Sarah H.
    Swift Foundation, Inc.
Mr. Larry Korman
McNeil Pharmaceutical
Phillips Foundation
Sandoz, Inc.
Smith Kline Beckman Corporation
Tappanz Foundation, Inc.
The Upjohn Company
van Amerigen Foundation, Inc.
Wyeth Laboratories
Mr. and Mrs. William A. Zales